THE FULL DIET

Dr Saira Hameed is one of the UK's leading weight-loss doctors. She is a Consultant Endocrinologist at the NHS Imperial Weight Centre, an internationally renowned centre of excellence for weight management, and a Senior Tutor and Honorary Clinical Senior Lecturer at Imperial College London. Dr Hameed read medicine at Oxford University and University College London, and received her PhD on the body's control of weight and appetite from Imperial College London. Through her work in the NHS and Imperial College, Dr Hameed created Imperial-SatPro, the highly effective, often life-changing, weight-loss programme on which *The Full Diet* is based. Dr Hameed lives in London with her family. *The Full Diet* is her first book.

The Full Diet

DR SAIRA HAMEED

MICHAEL 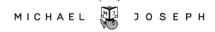 JOSEPH

MICHAEL JOSEPH

UK | USA | Canada | Ireland | Australia
India | New Zealand | South Africa

Michael Joseph is part of the Penguin Random House group of companies
whose addresses can be found at global.penguinrandomhouse.com

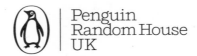

First published by Michael Joseph, 2022
003

Copyright © Dr Saira Hameed, 2022

The moral right of the author has been asserted

Set in 12.5pt/16pt Garamond MT
Typeset by Couper Street Type Co.
Printed in Great Britain by Clays Ltd, Elcograf S.p.A.

The authorized representative in the EEA is Penguin Random House Ireland,
Morrison Chambers, 32 Nassau Street, Dublin D02 YH68

A CIP catalogue record for this book is available from the British Library

ISBN: 978-0-241-55245-2

www.greenpenguin.co.uk

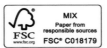

MIX
Paper from
responsible sources
FSC® C018179

Penguin Random House is committed to a
sustainable future for our business, our readers
and our planet. This book is made from Forest
Stewardship Council® certified paper.

For Jonathan

Contents

CONTENTS

INTRODUCTION

Every year thousands of scientific discoveries are made about weight loss, exercise, sleep, brain function and behaviour change. Yet most people who seek help with their weight are not told about this powerful new science. Instead of serving the people that need to hear about it the most, these cutting-edge breakthroughs stay in the laboratories and scientific journals.

This book will change that.

The Full Diet is based on this game-changing science – a pioneering, multi-dimensional programme that gets exceptional weight-loss results.

Designed by me and my colleagues – doctors and scientists at Imperial College London – The Full Diet was born out of the question: 'What if . . . ?'

'What if we shared the science with our patients?'

'What if we could create a weight-loss programme so well crafted, accessible and enjoyable that our patients could benefit from the transformative force of this great science?'

We carefully examined the scientific evidence, combined it with our clinical expertise, and we built a new weight-loss programme.

After other medical and scientific experts had reviewed the programme, we asked our patients at the Imperial Weight Centre – one of the UK's leading NHS weight-loss clinics – if they wanted to try something new. They did, with many taking part in a clinical research study of The Full Diet. The results, which we published in a leading scientific journal, show that a programme that follows the science gets outstanding results. Our patients typically lose a similar amount of weight to people who have had gastric band surgery. They also see their blood pressure fall, their diabetes reverse and their happiness and wellbeing sky-rocket.

With the research results now in, The Full Diet (which I also call the Programme in this book) was helping more and more people in our NHS clinic to lose weight. As news of the Programme's remarkable weight-loss outcomes spread, it became clear that no matter how many people I saw, there were many more who could benefit. That's why I decided to write this book. By reading these chapters, you will find out everything that my patients learn, so that its winning formula can work for you too.

The Full Diet can help anyone, however much weight you want to lose – from a few pounds to several stone. Once you know the science of how your body works and how to build a more comfortable and contented inner life, you can use these universal tools for living life at a weight that's right for you.

Unlike restrictive diets that leave you feeling unsatisfied, at its heart The Full Diet harnesses the filling power of your body's hunger and fullness system so that it works in harmony with your weight-loss goals. If you take a look at the recipes on pages 219–89, you can see that you will be eating well. These delicious food choices will also make you feel full, allowing you to effortlessly stop eating when your body has had enough – there's no willpower required, just science. You will now be working *with* your body's biology – forming a partnership that's pulling in the same direction – to lose weight and live life to the full.

You will also find, like many of my patients, that the results of The Full Diet go far beyond weight loss. From improving sleep and getting the buzz of exercise to feeling more energetic and building greater self-compassion, the Programme has a powerful whole-life ripple effect. This is reflected in the book's title, *The Full Diet*, chosen not only for its physical fullness effects but also because the Programme addresses and fills up emotional hunger, reframing how you care for and value yourself as the precious human being you are.

All you need is a sense of curiosity about how your brilliant body works, and an open mind about the practical strategies that have helped so many others before you to feel good and lose weight.

Welcome to The Full Diet: your healthier, happier, fuller future is just about to begin.

HOW TO USE THIS BOOK

The content of the chapters in this book mirrors the fortnightly Programme sessions that my patients attend as a group. Just like these chapters, our sessions are fizzing with science, information and know-how. From looking after your gut bacteria to understanding your brain's inner workings, our sessions are as gripping as watching a great box set or series – my patients often say, 'I can't wait to find out what happens next!'

This is exactly as it should be; central to the Programme's design is the idea that science is exciting, especially when we ask what it can do for us in our everyday lives. It's this wealth of practical strategies – your Programme tools – that are the big reveal at the end of each session or chapter. Your tools are your Programme changes, that will take you to your weight-loss success. Using a particular tool is not a 'rule' – there are no 'rules' in the Programme. Instead, you have choices. The science is your guide to why a choice or tool is being recommended. You can then decide whether it feels right for you and your own situation. It's your Programme and you are in control.

Similarly, you can choose the pace at which you want to read this book. You might prefer to read it cover to cover and then get started. Alternatively, you can pause at the end of each chapter and get up and running with your newest tool before moving on to the next one. Whatever suits you best is the right answer. This is not a sprint to an imaginary finish line. Instead, it's a process of long-term lifestyle change that you will find becomes richer and more rewarding as you continue to move forward.

Everyone I look after in the Programme has a medical consultation ahead of taking part. Before you begin The Full Diet, please discuss it with your doctor (see page 294). If, after reviewing your health background and any medication you are taking, you both agree that the Programme is a great fit for you, then you are ready to get started.

So here we are, at one of my favourite Programme moments. In our patient groups, it's the buzz of anticipation in the room just before the first session begins. Or in our case, being a moment away from starting Chapter 1. Having seen the life-changing effects of the Programme in my patients, I am excited that the same possibilities lie ahead for you. I wish I could be with you in person, but instead, like a coach on the touchline, I am cheering you on every step of the way.

CHAPTER I

Food

'I used to suffer from high blood pressure, type
2 diabetes and high cholesterol. The emphasis
is on "used to". I have now reversed my high
blood pressure and diabetes and I have stopped
taking medication that I was told I would be on
for life. So what did I change? I was educated on
how my body actually works and on using food
as my medicine, and that's exactly what I did.'
Anil, lost 4 stone 10lb (30kg)

Imagine you had been given a state-of-the-art sports car. As
the owner of this elegant piece of machinery you would have
some choices to make about how to treat it. Would you service
it, clean it, take care when driving and use the very best fuel
available to keep it running in top condition? Or would you
drive it into the ground, park it bumper to bumper, never take
it to the garage and put in whatever fuel you could find, even
if that fuel damaged the engine and made the car break down?

The answer might seem obvious, but the interesting thing
is that while we instinctively look after material possessions

that we consider valuable, like an expensive car, we can often relegate the care of our body – which is, after all, infinitely more precious – to an afterthought. This is an approach that will not work in the long term because while your possessions are replaceable, your body is not.

To continue the analogy, if you put diesel into a petrol car, it won't run well. Yet every day, many of us put the wrong fuel into our bodies, and when the body responds with howls of protest – in the form of bloating, acid reflux, headaches, fatigue, low mood, poor sleep and weight gain – we ignore the message. Petrol cars don't run well on diesel. In the same way, you can't fuel your body with 'food' that it doesn't recognize as food and expect to feel good – or be the weight you want to be.

In this chapter, you will learn the science that explains why the foods that you have been eating are preventing you from losing weight and you'll come away knowing which foods are the right fuel for your body. Like my patient Anil, whose inspiring words open the chapter, you will see how food can be your medicine and you too can choose to eat in a way that gives you a powerful prescription for losing weight, regaining your health and feeling good.

Insulin: the fat controller

All food is made up of small building blocks. The building block of carbohydrates – foods like bread, pasta, rice and breakfast cereal – is a sugar called glucose. When you eat these foods, your body quickly breaks them down into the component sugar (glucose) building blocks, which move from your gut into your blood. If you have two pieces of toast, a bowl of cornflakes and a glass of orange juice for breakfast, the increase in your blood sugar level will be equivalent to 24 teaspoons of sugar. By the time that sugar has hit your blood, your body has no idea whether you have had toast, cereal and juice for breakfast or a slice of cake – the effect on your blood sugar level is the same.

If carbohydrate foods make up a large proportion of your daily diet (see the Choose Not to Eat List on pages 24–5) and perhaps you eat cereal and toast for breakfast, a sandwich and juice for lunch and pasta for dinner – a diet often considered completely normal – you will have consumed a large amount of sugar that day, maybe the equivalent of more than 40 teaspoons. For context: the body needs the equivalent of 1 teaspoon in the blood at any one time to function well.

Your body does not like to have this extra sugar in the blood because it disturbs its natural equilibrium, interfering with its correct functioning. So to remove this excess sugar from the blood, and to bring the blood sugar level back down to normal, the body produces a hormone called insulin.

I like to think of insulin as being like a janitor managing your blood sugar level with a broom. Insulin will sweep excess sugar – from foods like bread, rice, potatoes and cereal – out of your blood, but insulin can't make the sugar magically disappear. Instead, insulin will sweep any sugar that is not immediately needed for use by your body into storage. Insulin can sweep a small amount of sugar into your liver and your muscles but your liver and muscles have a limited storage capacity. Once they are full, any excess sugar must be stored somewhere else. So insulin sweeps this remaining sugar into your fat.

This means that the more bread, rice, pasta, potatoes, crackers, cereal, crisps and biscuits that you eat, the more sugar will end up in your blood and the more insulin will be sweeping, all the time, to store that sugar as fat. The result is that you gain weight.

My patients find this core Programme concept really sticks in their memory when we give our insulin janitor a job title: insulin is 'the fat controller'.

In my experience, my patients resolutely want to follow the dietary advice that they are given. When I first meet them, they describe eating cereal for breakfast, a sandwich at lunch and pasta for dinner, just as they have been told to do, yet they continue to put on weight. You can now see why.

This way of eating is a high-sugar diet and most of this sugar will be swept into fat by insulin, the fat controller. Eating these sorts of foods makes you a very efficient fat-storing machine.

The Programme helps you to break this cycle by instead choosing to eat delicious, natural, low-sugar foods that will transform you into a fat-burning machine.

How does this happen? Well, when you eat foods like eggs and vegetables and yogurt and nuts that are not made of sugar building blocks, very little sugar ends up in your blood after eating. This means your body doesn't need to produce much insulin to sweep excess sugar out of your blood and into fat. Better still, low insulin levels are a signal to your fat to break itself down – and when fat is broken down, you lose weight.

Getting off the blood sugar rollercoaster

If up until now you have been eating a high-carbohydrate diet (cereal, sandwiches, pasta, biscuits, crisps and juice), then a large amount of sugar will end up in your blood after eating. This surge in your blood sugar level will be abruptly followed by a sugar crash as insulin does its job, sweeping that sugar out of your blood and into fat storage. These big swings in your blood sugar level disrupt your body's equilibrium; and one part of your body in particular finds a sudden sugar high, followed by a crashing low, especially hard to deal with: your brain.

The rapid change in blood sugar level from high to low can make you feel grumpy, foggy and lethargic. Since this is an unpleasant way to feel, you then seek out more sugar to counteract the sugar low. So you eat three biscuits mid-morning, which are quickly broken down into the equivalent of 12 more teaspoons of sugar, giving you another blood sugar high.

Temporarily your brain feels a bit better, but then suddenly insulin has once again swept that sugar into fat. Blood sugar levels drop and you feel tired and irritable. So you decide to go for an early lunch of a sandwich, a packet of crisps and a bottle of juice – that's the equivalent of 18 more teaspoons of sugar . . . and so the blood-sugar rollercoaster ride goes on.

The good news is that your Programme food choices give you your exit pass off the blood-sugar rollercoaster. Foods that form the basis of the Programme are deliberately chosen because they do not cause a surge in your blood sugar followed by a crashing low. By eating foods like fish, nuts, cheese, meat, fruit, eggs and vegetables, the Programme stabilizes your blood sugar level and this will make you feel good. Your mood will feel brighter and your energy levels will soar.

The age-old wisdom of eating fat

For tens of thousands of years, human beings have eaten fat in the way nature provides it – as golden egg yolks, the marbling through a cut of meat, the refreshing white flesh of a coconut and the verdant green of olive oil.

Forty years ago, food guidelines were issued based on the idea that eating fat was the cause of cardiovascular diseases such as heart attacks and was also responsible for weight gain. Fat, an ancient foodstuff, eaten by humans for millennia, was now being blamed for modern disease epidemics.

Recently, the evidence behind the 'eat low-fat' guidance has been questioned, but even at the time the advice was subject to heated debate. The misgivings of many in the scientific community about the low-fat advice were summed up in 1980 by Dr Philip Handler, the then President of the US National Academy of Sciences, who asked, 'What right has the government to propose that the American people conduct a vast nutritional experiment, with themselves as subjects, on the strength of so little evidence that it will do them any good?'

Nevertheless, low-fat became synonymous with healthy eating and millions of people cut fat out of their diet. Full-fat creamy whole milk was switched to low-fat skimmed. The skin was dutifully cut off the Sunday roast chicken and left untouched on the side of the plate. Thick natural yogurt was rejected in favour of low-fat varieties that had to be bulked out with starches and sweeteners to make them edible. Margarine, which, until the mid-twentieth century, had been mandated by law in certain US states to be dyed pink or other offputting colours to indicate it was an unnatural food, now became the 'healthy' choice.

Food surveys, such as the annual report carried out by DEFRA (the Department for Environment, Food and Rural Affairs), show that the public was responsibly following the 'eat low-fat' advice, but an alarming trend was emerging. While we were replacing the foods of our grandparents with anything that was labelled 'low-fat' or 'light', the nation was getting fatter.

In 1980, just before the low-fat guidance was issued, 7 per cent of the country were, by medical classification, obese, a condition that now affects more than one in four of us. When we also include the number of people who are over-weight, we see that 64 per cent of us have a weight issue, which means that in the UK today it is more 'normal' to be overweight or obese than to live at a healthy body weight. Yet we know that people are following the guidelines and doing what they have been told is the right thing.

Interestingly, traditional cultures around the world that were not asked to follow dietary guidelines and instead

continued to eat in the way their ancestors had for generations – including dietary fat – remained lean, while we gritted
our teeth, cut out the fat and became heavier.

In the past, before dietary guidelines, we had followed a
food culture. We learnt about cooking, food and eating from
our parents and grandparents. Each society had its own food
wisdom that had served it well for hundreds, even thousands of years. The food guidelines changed this; they called
into question the way of eating that had been learnt through
family ties and made us unsure of ourselves.

This opened up a whole new market for the food industry,
and ultra-processed foods promising us 'low-fat', 'fat-free'
and 'light' proliferated on supermarket shelves. The problem of the unpleasant taste and watery consistency when fat
is taken out of food was circumvented by adding in starches,
thickeners and sugar to make low-fat food more palatable.

If you look in your kitchen today, I am almost certain
that you will find some or all of the following: skimmed
or semi-skimmed milk, diet yogurts, margarine or low-fat
spreads, no-fat cooking spray, reduced-fat mayonnaise, skinless chicken breasts, low-fat ready meals and a variety of tins
and boxes declaring their health benefits because of the lack
of fat inside them.

When you look at this food in its bright packaging covered
in health promises, do you look forward to eating it? Does
a diet yogurt satisfy you, or as the spoon hits the bottom of
the pot are you already thinking, 'What's next?' If you ran out
of milk and had to add water to your tea instead of skimmed
milk, would you genuinely notice a taste difference?

So why should you eat fat?

Firstly, it tastes delicious. Wouldn't you rather eat the crispy skin as well as the roast chicken or sauté your vegetables in butter rather than eating them with a low-fat dressing?

Secondly, fat is satisfying. People who come to my clinic describe how, after eating a low-fat yogurt, they are still hungry, but there is a limit to how much thick, creamy Greek yogurt you can eat because it is a food containing natural fats, so it makes you feel full. Feeling full is an important part of why Programme eating feels so good.

Lastly, eating certain fats, such as those found in olive oil and nuts, has health benefits, including reducing the risk of a heart attack or stroke. In one landmark clinical trial, participants were divided into three groups. One group ate a low-fat diet while the other two groups ate a Mediterranean diet supplemented with either olive oil or nuts. The cardiovascular health benefits of these fats were demonstrated so clearly that the study was stopped early – the much higher rate of heart attacks and strokes in the low-fat diet group meant that it was considered unethical to continue the trial.

Eating fat does not make you fat

At this stage, my patients will frequently ask me, 'If I eat fat, won't I get fat?' I am always pleased to reassure them that the answer is 'no'. As we saw at the beginning of this chapter, sugar makes us fat; naturally occurring fats in meat, fish, olive oil, dairy, nuts and seeds do not. It is simply an unfortunate slip of the English language that we use the same word for the 'fat' in food and 'fat' in the body. In fact, the correct medical word for body fat is 'adipose tissue'. In order to get away from the idea that eating fat must make you fat, start thinking of body fat as 'adipose tissue', which will reinforce to you that 'fat' in food and 'fat' in the body are two totally different things, an etymological coincidence resulting in decades of confusion.

What about my cholesterol?

The second question I am often asked is, 'If I eat fat, won't my cholesterol increase?' This is an understandable worry because of the idea that the fats we eat 'fur up' the arteries, which could lead to a heart attack or stroke.

The cholesterol that is measured in your blood tests is not the cholesterol that you eat but is actually made inside your body by your liver; it has almost nothing to do with how much cholesterol you are or aren't eating. In fact, the latest US government dietary guidelines have now removed previously advised limits on dietary cholesterol consumption.

I can also reassure my patients about their cholesterol because in both our research study as well as in our clinic, by following the Programme our patients' cholesterol blood tests improve. Although they are now eating and enjoying a wealth of natural healthy fats, there is an increase in their 'good, heart-healthy' (HDL) cholesterol as well as a fall in their triglyceride levels. Triglycerides are fatty particles in the blood linked to metabolic syndrome, a condition associated with a high risk of heart attacks and strokes. So with lower triglyceride levels, my patients have reduced their risk of developing these diseases. And my patients achieve these improvements in their cholesterol blood tests despite clearing their kitchens of low-fat foods and instead eating the same delicious fats that their grandparents did.

What would Grandma do?

When your grandma made her roast chicken with buttered vegetables, she didn't have to read a food label or refer to an app to check if this was a healthy meal. What she knew was that she was making the same roast chicken that her mother before her had made, that it tasted good and the family loved eating it. This food wisdom, which had made eating a straightforward business, has now been superseded by confusion and worry. This is because food has become unnecessarily complicated. Instead of eating what is clearly food – such as chicken, fish, eggs, nuts, carrots and strawberries – we are eating food with long lists of ingredients, which are so far removed from what has been eaten through most of human history that sometimes it is not clear to your body whether you are actually eating food at all.

To illustrate this point, at Session 1 I ask my patients if, simply based on the ingredients, they could identify what this is:

Wheat Flour, Sugar, Soya Bean and Palm Oil (Antioxidant (E319)), Glucose Fructose Syrup, Dextrose, Glucose Syrup, Chocolate Chips (7.2%) (Sugar, Chocolate Powder, Dextrose, Cocoa Butter, Soy Lecithin, Milk, Vanilla Extract), Wheat Flour, Salt, Modified Food Starch, Raising Agents (E500, E541), Natural Colour (E150a), Milk Gelatine (from Beef), Thickener (E481), Food Starch, Stabilizer (E472e), Natural and Artificial Flavourings, Xanthan Gum, Egg Whites, Soy Lecithin, Artificial Colours (E129, E110, E102, E132)

They could not, although one of my patients gave the inspired answer, 'Diabetes in a packet!'

In fact, it's a chocolate-chip flavoured toaster pastry, although, for our purposes, it doesn't really matter what this food is. It could be industrially produced biscuits, a frozen dessert or a coffee-shop muffin, but if your brain does not understand the ingredients, don't expect the packet to contain fuel that your body wants to use.

In general, our grandparents did not eat foods like this and they lived at a healthy weight, free from diabetes and other health problems. Over the past few decades, we have been led down a different path, which has taken us to a place where we don't want to be. Either we need to 'try harder' with the dubious ingredients and complicated labelling, or we might choose to conclude that generations of food wisdom is unlikely to have been wrong. Instead, by going back to eating the foods that humans are designed to eat, we can live free of weight problems, just as our grandparents did.

CHOICES

The way the Programme works is that once you know the science, you can choose if you want to use it to lose weight and improve your health. The choices at the end of each chapter give you a practical way to apply the science of how your body works, so that you are working with your biology to achieve your weight-loss goals.

Choice 1: Choose to fuel your body with foods that turn you into a fat-burning machine

The Full Diet only ever involves eating real, nourishing, natural food. There are no supplements or meal replacements. There is no counting, weighing or measuring of food. You can shop at your usual supermarket and continue to enjoy eating out in restaurants and at social occasions. And you will be doing all of this in the knowledge that you are looking after your body, giving it the right fuel so that it runs well and you feel good.

Before you look through the list below, it's important to bear in mind that the foods you will be choosing to eat on the Programme are far more plentiful, delicious and varied than the foods you are choosing not to eat. It is simply that the foods you will be choosing not to eat have, over the last few decades, come to dominate the Western diet. This has given the false impression that they are necessary or essential. In fact, these are the very foods that are not working for you and are keeping you at a weight that you don't want to be.

On the Programme you eat food that does not break down into a lot of sugar. This will keep your insulin levels low. Low insulin levels are the signal to fat to break down, so you lose weight – these foods, on your **Choose to Eat List**, make you an efficient fat-burning machine:

FRUIT AND VEGETABLES

- All vegetables (except for potatoes and other starchy vegetables, such as parsnips and sweet potatoes)
- Vegetables (can be fresh or frozen) – examples include: baby corn, broccoli, Brussels sprouts, cabbage, carrots, cauliflower, celeriac, garlic, green or runner beans, kale, mushrooms, onions and spinach
- Salad veg, such as celery, cucumber, radishes, lettuce and other green salad leaves
- Fruit-like vegetables, including avocados, aubergines, courgettes, peppers and tomatoes
- Lemons and limes
- Low- and medium-sugar fruit, such as apples, pears, blueberries, raspberries and strawberries (fruit is naturally sweet and contains sugar, so it's best not to overdo it – you could, for example, choose an apple one day, a handful of berries the next)

EGGS

DAIRY

- Whole, full-fat milk (up to 100ml or so per day)

- Natural (plain) or Greek full-fat yogurt (up to about 200g per day)
- Kefir (check it only has two ingredients – milk and beneficial bacteria cultures)
- Cheese, such as Cheddar, feta, halloumi, mozzarella, Parmesan and cream cheese (about 100g per day)
- Cream – single, double or clotted (about 2 tablespoons per day)
- Crème fraîche – full-fat (about 2 tablespoons per day)
- Butter – salted or unsalted, depending on your preference
- Non-dairy milk alternatives (check the ingredients are straightforward – for example, almond milk should only contain almonds, water and sometimes sea salt)

MEAT

- Any kind of fresh meat – for example, beef, chicken, lamb, pork and turkey (check there's no breading, sauces or dubious ingredients and that it's just a one-ingredient food – meat!)
- Bacon
- Sausages – pork, beef, chicken or lamb with a high meat content, which means more than 90 per cent meat
- Sliced ham or turkey (check there's no added sugar, honey, syrups or breading)
- Antipasto selection – for example, prosciutto and salami
- Pâté (check there's no added sugar and it only contains pronounceable ingredients)

FISH

- Any fish and shellfish, fresh or frozen (but not in breading, batter or sauces; it should be just one ingredient – fish!)

GENERAL

- Dips, such as hummus, tzatziki and guacamole
- Pesto

- Full-fat mayonnaise (check that the ingredients are straightforward and sound like food)
- Mustard (steer clear of any that list ingredients that you wouldn't keep in your kitchen)
- Vinegar, such as white wine vinegar or apple cider vinegar
- Olives
- Tofu
- Cooking fats – olive oil, lard, coconut oil and ghee
- Fresh and dried herbs and spices
- Raw unsalted nuts, including almonds, Brazil nuts, macadamias, pecans, pistachios and walnuts (about a handful per day – check there are no added ingredients, like a honey glaze)
- Nut butters, such as peanut butter and almond butter (about 2 teaspoons per day – check there is no added sugar)
- Seeds, such as flaxseed (also known as linseed), hemp seeds, pumpkin seeds, sesame seeds and sunflower seeds (a handful or two per day)
- Legumes, including lentils, beans (not baked beans) and chickpeas (up to one serving per day)
- Long-life tomato foods, like passata, tomato purée, tinned tomatoes and sundried tomatoes
- Good-quality dark chocolate – 85% or 90% cocoa solids
- Water – still or sparkling (but not flavoured or sweetened waters)
- Herbal or fruit tea – for example, camomile or mint
- Coffee – not with lots of milk (avoid a latte or flat white and please don't add syrups or sugar)
- Tea, including green tea (again, no added sugar)

The best way to get an idea of what your day will look like eating these foods is to have a look at the sample Programme menu on page 290, as well as the recipes that start on page 219 – you will see some delicious and amazingly good eating awaits you.

Even though there is no calorie counting (see page 39), this is not an all-you-can-eat plan (see pages 209–10). So the mindset here is to apply common sense, which I know you will. For example, an omelette for one person is made of two or maybe three eggs, not six, and an avocado serving is half or one, not three. Look at the portion sizes on the food list and the number of servings in the recipes for guidance and, most importantly, choose to stop eating when you are full (there's lots more about this in Chapters 2 and 14).

In time, as you get further into the Programme and start to feel its benefits, you might choose to tailor your eating to your specific tastes, preferences and lifestyle by introducing some other foods that are not on this list. There's lots of information about how to do this on pages 117–9 and 201–2. If you do choose to adapt the food list, I'd encourage you to continue to fuel your body with natural wholefoods, steering clear of processed foods with dubious ingredients, and I'd suggest mostly sticking to the Choose to Eat List because of all the inbuilt weight-loss and health benefits. However, occasionally you might choose to eat a slice of homemade cake at a family birthday party or some bread at a special restaurant meal.

When we discuss this in our groups, I advise my patients to use the food lists as written until they are fully into their Programme stride, to minimize the chance of any off-list food causing them to backtrack. I also advise that they hold off any reintroductions until they are close to or at the weight they want to be. This means that if a food stalls their weight loss or even results in weight gain, it causes less of a dent in their momentum. This Programme is for you and in time you will get a feel for how you can shape it to your needs so that, like my many successful patients who have lost weight and reclaimed their health, it becomes your lifelong way of eating.

Choice 2: Choose not to eat foods that make you an efficient fat-storage machine

The foods listed below are broken down into sugar by your body, which ends up in your blood. As you know, insulin (the fat controller) will then get to work sweeping the excess sugar into fat storage.

So to keep your insulin level low, here's your **Choose Not to Eat List**:

- Bread of any kind, including sliced, bagels, baguettes, chapatti, ciabatta, flatbreads, naan, pitta, rolls, tortillas and wraps
- Pasta
- Rice
- Couscous
- Noodles
- Breakfast cereals, including oats/porridge, muesli and granola
- Cereal bars
- Crackers
- Potatoes, including crisps and chips
- Baked goods, including biscuits, brownies, cakes, croissants, flapjacks, muffins and pastries

- Pizza
- Pastry (sweet or savoury)
- Sweets and chocolates
- Ice cream, sorbets and ice lollies
- Jam, marmalade and other sugar-based spreads
- Sugar, honey and syrups
- Artificial sweeteners
- High-sugar fruits, such as bananas, mangoes, grapes and pineapple
- Dried fruit
- Fruit juice (no matter how healthy the labelling claims)
- Smoothies (shop-bought or homemade)
- Squash drinks
- Fizzy drinks (including diet or no-calorie versions)
- Ketchup and other high-sugar condiments, such as barbecue sauce
- Shop-bought salad dressings
- Shop-bought sauces and stir-in cooking sauces
- Ready meals

When we look at this food list at Session 1, some of my patients initially worry or are even alarmed at the idea of stepping away from certain foods. Perhaps you feel that way too. The reality is, however you decide to reinvigorate your health and lose weight, you will need to make some changes in order to achieve your goal. Even people who have bariatric (weight-loss) surgery have to follow a specific life-long eating plan after the operation, otherwise they will regain weight.

Putting some restrictions on the food that you eat will not take anything away from you; in fact, these restrictions will end up setting you free. As my patients often tell me, eating in an unrestricted way was restricting other areas of their life, for example affecting their confidence, mood or health. Instead, when they joined the Programme and chose to eat with a few restrictions, this became their gateway to an unrestricted life.

Choice 3: Choose to eat natural, healthy fats and to avoid synthetic, processed fats

Broadly speaking, there are two sorts of fats. The first are fats that nature put on the planet for us, such as those found in dairy, meat, oily fish, nuts, seeds, natural oils like olive oil and certain wholefoods, such as avocados. If you choose to eat fat in the way that nature has provided it, you won't go wrong.

The second category of fats are industrially produced fats, such as trans fats, which are linked to illnesses like cardiovascular disease and which play no part in the Programme. We also keep away from anything that has been engineered to be 'low-fat'.

Choose to eat fats that nature put on the planet to nourish you	Choose to avoid highly processed oils and artificial trans fats
Olive oil	Highly processed vegetable (seed) oils, such as corn oil, sunflower oil and palm oil
Butter	Artificial trans fats
Ghee	'Low-fat' cooking sprays
Lard or dripping	Vegetable shortening

Coconut oil	Margarine and other low-fat spreads
Nuts, nut butters and seeds	Ultra-processed fried foods
Full-fat dairy, such as milk, yogurt and cheese	Shop-bought ultra-processed foods like crisps, biscuits, pastries and cakes
Fats found in natural, one-ingredient foods, such as avocados, oily fish and meat	Any product labelled low-fat, diet or light/lite

The Programme is not a 'high-fat' way of eating. Rather, it is about eating fat in the way that generations of humans always used to, enjoying it for its flavour, texture and filling qualities, as well as for its health benefits. This means cooking with fat in the same way your grandparents would have done, so butter on steamed vegetables means a teaspoon, not a pat. And we only add fat to food in a way that taps into a recognizable food culture, so a splash of full-fat milk in coffee, not oil or half a pot of cream.

Choice 4: Choose not to eat ultra-processed food that contains dubious ingredients

In our groups we emphasize this idea by imagining a scenario in which you visit a doctor. The doctor gives you some pills in a box that lists numerous unfamiliar chemical ingredients that neither you nor the doctor can pronounce. When you ask what these ingredients are, the doctor says, 'I don't know', but tells you to expect side-effects of bloating, indigestion, fatigue, headaches, sleep disruption, low mood and weight gain. Hearing this, I think it's unlikely that you would agree to take the pills. Yet it is now considered normal to eat ultra-processed foods, full of unpronounceable ingredients that we don't understand and that have similar side-effects to our medication example.

In The Full Diet, we avoid ultra-processed foods containing ingredients we don't recognize (there's lots more about this in Chapters 2, 7, 8 and 13). These ingredients are not the right fuel for your body – they belong in a chemistry lab, not inside you. Your grandparents wouldn't recognize these as foods and nor should you. As a rule of thumb, if you don't understand what an ingredient is, don't eat it.

Choice 5: Choose not to eat artificial sweeteners

Artificial sweeteners play no part in the Programme. This includes artificial sweeteners added to tea or coffee, used in recipes, and included in diet drinks and any pre-prepared food.

Why is this?

First, the clue is in the name – artificial. This Programme is about real, natural, nourishing food. No chemicals. No tricks.

Secondly, artificial sweeteners increase insulin levels, putting you into fat-storage mode. This is because the sugary taste of artificial sweeteners tricks your body into thinking that sugar is on its way and, in anticipation of this, the body produces insulin pre-emptively. Since you know that insulin is the fat-storage hormone (the fat controller), you can see why, despite the 'zero-calorie' promises, artificial sweeteners will not help with weight loss.

Thirdly, although artificial sweeteners taste sugary, because they are chemically different from sugar, sweeteners do not satisfy sweet cravings, which can result in overeating as the body seeks out further sweet foods to compensate.

Lastly, it is only by removing overly sweet tastes from your food that you can recalibrate your body's perception of natural sweetness. If you use artificial sweeteners, this readjustment won't happen and foods that are not overly and unnaturally sweet will taste bland. Your habit of expecting food to taste exceptionally sweet will continue. Once weaned from this unnatural sweetness, you will start to appreciate the natural sugars in many foods – the fresh sweetness of a carrot, the velvety taste of Greek yogurt, the richness of 90% cocoa chocolate.

So you can see that while foods and soft drinks containing artificial sweeteners make promises like 'zero calories', you now know that there's actually no such thing as a free lunch.

Choice 6: Choose to be cautious with alcohol

Alcohol is a high-sugar drink. Some alcoholic drinks are lower in sugar than others – for instance, red wine is less sugary than beer – but all alcohol is a fermented sugar solution.

Alcohol will affect your Programme progress because sugar in alcohol equals sugar in the blood equals insulin – the fat controller – sweeping that sugar into fat, which equals weight gain.

Alcohol also has a number of other unwanted effects.

First, it lowers resolve and makes you feel hungry, so you are far more likely to make off-Programme food choices when you are drinking.

Secondly, alcohol destabilizes your blood sugar level, causing it to rise and then quickly fall. As you know, The Full Diet aims to move you away from this blood-sugar rollercoaster, so your blood sugar stays steady – and you feel good.

Thirdly, alcohol is a sleep disruptor. You might feel that you sleep soundly after drinking, but in fact your sleep will have been of poor quality. Sleep is important to your weight and your health (see Chapter 6). Disturbed, poor-quality sleep results in high insulin levels the next day – in other words, it puts you in fat-storing mode. Poor sleep also results in hunger hormones running high, which means that the day after drinking you will be hungrier.

Finally, rather than relieving stress, alcohol itself causes stress. If you feel you need alcohol to deal with stress or to unwind, this could be an issue that you might want to discuss with your GP.

For all of these reasons, be cautious with alcohol and choose not to drink for the first eight weeks of the Programme, while you are developing your new routine.

Some of my patients have worried that friends and family will respond negatively if they choose not to drink alcohol. In fact, more and more people are reducing their alcohol intake or are deciding on a period of abstinence for health reasons, so you will find that you aren't unusual within a group. Many of my patients have also discovered that after a few social occasions of choosing not to drink alcohol, sparkling water with ice and lemon became their 'thing' – and then because it was their 'thing', it was just automatically ordered or poured for them by their friends without comment.

Once you are up and running in the Programme, you might choose to reintroduce a small amount of alcohol. But for all of the reasons described, make it infrequent – meaning once or twice a week at the most, and definitely not every day. If you decide to have a drink, I encourage you to make it worth it. Worth it means choosing good-quality alcohol, for example, a wine someone has recommended or that you have been given as a gift. Make it special. Choose an occasion that matters. Consume alcohol thoughtfully and slowly. Drink with people who mean something to you, rather than on your own, and choose to drink only a small amount.

Choice 7: Choose to clean out your kitchen

There's no better day to start than today. This means taking control of your fridge and your food cupboards. When my patients come to their first session, I give them a bin bag to take home, to remind them where the old, health-sapping food belongs.

Don't feel guilty and think you should finish things up and then start the Programme: your body is not a dustbin. In fact, I'd love you to come away from reading this book with a heightened appreciation – even awe – for how extraordinary your body actually is.

Please don't think you'll keep the rice and the pasta and the ketchup and the ice cream just in case. If these things are not available to you, you'll be much more likely to stay on track.

Don't hold on to biscuits for when you have guests. If someone was giving up smoking they wouldn't keep a packet of cigarettes in the house just in case a friend came over and wanted one. You know this would be a very risky strategy. Instead, take pleasure from filling up the bin bag with foods that are not the right fuel for your body and that are stopping you from being the weight you want to be.

Choice 8: Choose to ask for support

If you live with other people, then enlist their support. In my experience, family members usually want to do everything they can to help. Explain to them that you have made an important commitment to a new, lifelong way of eating. That certain foods were not working for you and were affecting your health and weight. Don't feel bad about this. If you were allergic to peanuts, no one would insist on having peanut butter in the house just because they like to eat it. Instead, they would respect your health requirements and support you.

Even if other family members don't want to lose weight, they can still reap health and wellbeing benefits from enjoying delicious Programme food with you – and if you are doing this together, it becomes even more fun.

Choice 9: Choose to take it one day at a time

On day 1, 'the rest of my life' sounds like a very long time. Pause a moment.

All you need to do at this stage is commit to following The Full Diet today. Then tomorrow you can choose to follow the Programme again that day.

What you will find is that the food you are eating is delicious and filling and at the same time you will be losing weight and feeling so much better in yourself. Soon the decision to continue will stop being a daily choice and instead this new way of eating will become a natural and normal part of what you do and the way you live.

In the words of one of my patients, Tricia, who is three years in, 6 stone (38kg) lighter and going from strength to strength, 'The Programme is truly my life now and I will never ever change back.'

CHAPTER 2

Gut–brain signals

**'The Programme is as far from a diet as it
is possible to be – you always feel full and
have plenty of choices; you feel strong and
you never want to hear about going back
to your old eating habits. This is because
the Programme goes deeper: by explaining
the science as well as giving practical
advice, it holistically offers a new life.'**
Kostas, lost 2 stone 2lb (14kg)

Over hundreds of thousands of years, your body has evolved
a state-of-the-art, finely tuned hunger and fullness communication system between your gut and your brain. The
Programme has been designed around foods that fill you up
through their effect on this gut–brain communication.

If you currently feel confused about what hunger is or you
don't really know when you have eaten enough, then the science and the practical advice in this chapter will support you
to choose food that helps you to tune back into your body's
needs.

Unlike restrictive diets that you might have tried in the past, the Programme instead suggests being kind to your body and listening to its messages. This approach will transform your eating – allowing you to eat when you are hungry and stop when you are full. Eating will feel far more straightforward and you will lose weight and feel good.

Your body's brilliant
hunger–fullness signalling system

The hunger–fullness communication system between your gut and your brain is controlled by your body's hormones. You can think of hormones as being like your body's text messages, conveying important information from one part of your body to another.

When you haven't eaten for some time, your stomach sends out a hunger hormone signal called ghrelin. Ghrelin tells your brain, 'No fuel has come in for some time, I'm hungry. Find food.' The result of this communication between your gut and your brain is that you feel hungry. When you eat something, your stomach stops sending out the ghrelin hunger message, and so the feeling of hunger, which was there at the start of the meal, fades away.

On its own, turning down the ghrelin hunger signal is not enough to stop you eating. So when you eat, your gut sends out another hormone text message, this time about fullness. These fullness gut hormones (called glucagon-like peptide-1, peptide YY$_{3-36}$ and oxyntomodulin) tell your brain, 'Enough food has come in, you can stop eating now.' You experience this as the conscious thought, 'I'm done', or 'I'm finished with eating.'

Ultra-processed food breaks your hunger–fullness signalling system

Eat when you are hungry and stop when you are full is good eating advice but almost impossible to put into practice if you eat a lot of ultra-processed food. Your gut–brain communication has not been designed to know how to respond to the ingredients in these foods, which have only been eaten by humans for the last few decades.

If we go back to our example from Chapter 1 – how should your hunger and fullness system respond to these ingredients?

Wheat Flour, Sugar, Soya Bean and Palm Oil (Antioxidant (E319)), Glucose Fructose Syrup, Dextrose, Glucose Syrup, Chocolate Chips (7.2%) (Sugar, Chocolate Powder, Dextrose, Cocoa Butter, Soy Lecithin, Milk, Vanilla Extract), Wheat Flour, Salt, Modified Food Starch, Raising Agents (E500, E541), Natural Colour (E150a), Milk Gelatine (from Beef), Thickener (E481), Food Starch, Stabilizer (E472e), Natural and Artificial Flavourings, Xanthan Gum, Egg Whites, Soy Lecithin, Artificial Colours (E129, E110, E102, E132)

Your hunger and fullness hormones did not evolve to respond with any certainty to stabilizer (E472e) or soy lecithin. If you eat this food, should the hunger signal still be flashing? Perhaps the fullness signal should kick in? Or maybe, in a state of total confusion, you should be both hungry and full all at the same time?

Eating these ultra-processed foods results in chaos in the communication system (there's lots more about the devastating effect of these foods on our health in Chapter 8). It's the reason why, at the beginning of the Programme, my patients tell me, 'I'm not really certain what hunger is', or 'I'm always hungry', or 'I never seem to feel full no matter how much I eat.' Just as when a text message cannot get through and your phone display reads 'message failed to send', you are now in a gut-to-brain communication breakdown. There's been a hunger—fullness message failure.

But there is no need to worry. I can reassure you, as I do my patients, that the Programme will rebuild your gut—brain communication. When, like my patients, you turn your back on ultra-processed food and instead eat delicious, natural Programme food, the messages between your gut and brain will be rebooted and will start to come through loud and clear – and you will find it becomes easy to eat when you are hungry and stop when you are full, just as human beings were designed to do.

Leptin-brain communication

Your body stores energy in the form of body fat until it is needed to fuel your activities. The brain needs to know how much energy the body has stored, so body fat sends a hormone text message called leptin to the brain to keep it informed. When body fat stores are adequate, a leptin message goes to the brain to say, there's enough stored energy on board, there's no need to eat much.

If the amount of body fat increases further, the extra fat produces more of the leptin signal. When your body gets above a certain weight though, the fat-to-brain leptin message will become too loud and the brain tunes out. This breakdown in communication between energy stores (body fat) and the brain is called leptin resistance. Leptin resistance explains why it is possible to have a large amount of stored energy in the form of body fat and yet still feel hungry.

One cause of the breakdown of leptin-to-brain communication seems to be that too much insulin blocks the signalling system. The encouraging news is that by lowering your insulin levels through your food choices (Chapter 1), Eating Window (Chapter 3), exercise (Chapter 5) and getting enough sleep (Chapter 6), your insulin levels will fall and the leptin message will now get through to your brain. Your brain will hear that you have enough energy stored in body fat and the drive to eat is dialled down.

Why calorie counting doesn't work

The conventional approach to weight loss is to cut down the number of calories you are eating. This is the 'calories in, calories out' model, which supposes that if the amount you are eating (calories in) is less than the amount you are burning off (calories out), then you will lose weight. The flaw with this idea is its assumption that the human body is no more sophisticated than a car engine or a wood-burning stove. This is incorrect. Unlike a car or a stove, when you under-fuel your body, it mounts a powerful hormone counter-response to keep itself going.

Through hundreds of thousands of years of human evolution, the body has developed hardwired reactions to anything that threatens its survival, including food shortages. When you limit calories, your body has no idea that you are willingly doing this because you are on a weight-loss diet. Instead, the lack of food is registered as a survival threat – a warning of scarcity, even famine, ahead. This sets off a cascade of hormone changes known as the 'starvation response', which in the past bought us time so that we did not die (or at least not die immediately) when food was not available.

In response to semi-starvation (low-calorie dieting), your gut will produce the hunger hormone ghrelin, sending a text message to your brain to say, 'I'm hungry, find food.' This message will be repeatedly sent until you switch it off by eating something. Being hungry can make it hard to concentrate on anything else. You might feel irritable during the day and it's hard to fall asleep at night.

Gnawing, pit-of-the-stomach hunger, lack of concentration, short-temperedness and disrupted sleep make daily life on a low-calorie diet uncomfortable. This is compounded by feeling unsatisfied when you do eat because when incoming food is limited, your gut sends out a weaker fullness message after eating.

For a period of time you can be 'good' and use willpower to override the constant, uncomfortable hunger hormone signal as well as the lack of fullness after eating. After a while, though, these messages will be impossible to ignore and the diet will be broken. This is not about a lack of willpower, but all about your biology protecting you from the 'survival threat' of a low-calorie diet.

Turning down the thermostat – how low-calorie diets slow down your metabolism

Strong hunger signals and lack-of-fullness messages make low-calorie diets very difficult to stick to in the long term. But there's one more reason why calorie-restricted diets are destined to fail. Cutting calories generates hormone changes that slow down your metabolism.

Your metabolism is a term used to describe how your body uses fuel. We can think of metabolism as being like your central heating thermostat. If you wanted to use up fuel, you would turn up the thermostat. If you were short on fuel and wanted to conserve what you did have, then you would turn the thermostat down.

When you are on a low-calorie diet, there is less fuel coming in so your body turns down the thermostat (your metabolism) in order to use whatever fuel there is (the reduced amount of food) more efficiently.

A slowed-down metabolism in turn makes it hard for you to lose weight because it burns fewer calories, which is why you have to eat progressively less and less to keep your weight loss going.

A slow metabolism also doesn't feel good. A side-effect of your metabolism is heat production, so when your metabolism slows down on a low-calorie diet you feel cold. Your slowed metabolism will also make you feel tired and lacking in energy.

When wild animals go through periods of semi-starvation, they keep very still to conserve energy. They are certainly not wasting much-needed energy running the plains for leisure or jumping across the tree-tops to keep fit. In the same way, during calorie restriction your body shifts you towards stillness so as not to use up precious fuel unnecessarily. Your motivation to go to the gym or to go out for a walk falls to zero.

Now you understand how low-calorie diets trigger the starvation response and slow down your metabolism, I hope this helps you to stop blaming yourself for past restrictive diets that haven't worked. You can now see that low-calorie dieting puts you in an unrelenting fight with your body's bio-chemistry. When it's a question of willpower versus hundreds of thousands of years of human evolution, your biology will win every time.

Food is more than just calories

What low-calorie dieting means in practice is that food is chosen through the one-dimensional perspective of its calorie content. Low-calorie foods are 'good', higher-calorie foods are 'bad' and are to be avoided. The problem with this approach is that food is so much more than its calorie content. This is best demonstrated by the following example. On a low-calorie diet, you might eat a diet yogurt. The calorie content is 100 calories, which is just a drop in the ocean of your daily limit. Here are the ingredients:

Yogurt (Milk), Water, Fructose, Cocoa Butter, Cocoa Powder, Fat-reduced Cocoa Powder, Butter (Milk), Sugar, Modified Maize Starch, Gelatine; Stabilizers: Pectins, Guar Gum; Acidity Regulators: Citric Acid, Sodium Citrates, Calcium Citrates; Sweeteners: Aspartame, Acesulfame K; Flavourings: Carrot Juice Concentrate, Dark Chocolate Sprinkles (0.5%). Contains a source of Phenylalanine

Or you could choose to use those 100 calories and eat a boiled egg. Here are the ingredients:

Egg

From this example, you can clearly see that your body will respond to, digest, process and metabolize these two foods completely differently. The yogurt's high sugar content will mean that insulin is needed to sweep that sugar out of your blood and into fat storage. In contrast, the egg causes very little change in your blood sugar levels, which keeps insulin low. The sweetness of the diet yogurt will excite your brain's reward centre, resulting in cravings for more sweet things (more on this in Chapters 7, 8 and 13), whereas the egg, which does not taste sweet, will not. Artificial sweeteners in the 100-calorie yogurt will negatively affect the bacteria that live in your gut, which play a key role in regulating your weight and appetite (see Chapter 4). In contrast the protein content of the egg will tell your gut to release a strong fullness hormone signal, which messages your brain to say, 'That's enough, stop eating.' This is why no one comes to my clinic saying that once they start eating boiled eggs they just can't stop. Whereas a diet yogurt has you searching for the next thing to eat as soon as your spoon hits the bottom of the pot.

Two foods, with the same calorie content. But an egg is an egg and a diet yogurt is nineteen ingredients combined by food engineers to tick the 'low-calorie' box that shoppers are looking for. You now know that your body responds to food and not calories, which means that it is infinitely better to eat food, because when you eat food, your brilliant body takes care of the rest.

CHOICES

Now that you know the science of your hunger–fullness communication system, here's how you can use the power of these hormones to feel full and lose weight.

Choice 1: Choose to eat foods that turn up your gut-to-brain fullness signalling

Eating the kinds of food recommended in the Programme is the best way to encourage your gut to produce lots of fullness hormones. The Full Diet has been specifically designed to keep you feeling full!

Have a look back at the Choose to Eat List on pages 20–2. Eating these foods will give you lots of bang for your buck because not only are they delicious low-sugar foods that put you into fat-burning mode, these foods will also fill you up. Eating Programme foods will free you from restrictive diets that leave you unsatisfied and instead, after potentially years of fighting your body's biochemistry, you will now be working with your hormone signals.

Weight-loss operations like the gastric bypass work by increasing the strength of the gut's fullness hormones. There are also injectable fullness hormone medications that help people to lose weight. What's so brilliant is that your gut naturally makes lots of fullness hormones and by choosing to eat in a certain way, you can harness the power of your fullness hormones yourself to feel full and lose weight.

There are certain Programme foods that produce a particularly strong gut-to-brain fullness message. These are protein-rich foods that also contain healthy, natural fats. The strong fullness signal in response to eating protein is why sizzling lamb chops or grilled halloumi cheese are delicious, but it is rare to overeat these foods.

Protein-rich, fullness-boosting foods include eggs; meat; fish and shellfish; nuts and seeds; dairy, including milk, cream, Greek or natural yogurt and cheese; tofu, legumes and beans, such as chickpeas and lentils.

On the other hand, protein powders and shakes are not food and almost always contain artificial sweeteners and other dubious ingredients, so it's best to steer clear of them.

Please avoid going down the rabbit hole of thinking that if some protein is good, then more must be even better. I am certain that instead you will choose portions of protein that seem regular, so scrambled egg is two or three eggs, not six. Tuna mayo is one tin of tuna, not three. Although carbohydrates are high-sugar foods and require the most insulin to sweep that sugar out of the blood, you also produce insulin when you eat protein, so too much protein will similarly lead to weight gain.

The sample Programme menu on page 290 will give you an idea of what fullness eating looks like. Eating in this way is why, often for the first time in years, my patients get to the point in a meal when they feel the fullness hormone signal is strong and they stop eating – they know they have eaten enough. My patient Kostas, whose thoughtful words open the chapter, used the strength of these fullness messages to lose 2 stone 2lb (14kg) and reclaim his wellbeing. The Programme worked for Kostas because, unlike being on a restrictive low-calorie diet, 'you always feel full and have plenty of choices'. By tuning in to your body's fullness messages, these can be your words too.

Choice 2: Be patient!

Throughout this chapter, we have used the analogy of your fullness hormone signal being like a text message from your gut to your brain. There is, however, an important difference between a text and a hormone message. When you send a text, the recipient gets your message instantaneously. When your gut sends out a fullness hormone message after eating, it takes twenty minutes for your brain to get the information, 'You've eaten enough, you don't need to eat anything else.'

All smart restaurants know this, which is why, if you are offered the dessert menu as soon as your main course is cleared, it is likely you will order pudding. Whereas if service is slow and the waiter takes twenty minutes to ask you if you would like anything else to eat, your fullness signal will by then be strong and you are far more likely to say, 'No, thank you.'

So it's important to wait for twenty minutes after you finish eating before making a decision about whether you need to eat anything more. This break gives your fullness signal time to work. To get your eye in, you might want to set a timer on your phone. If after twenty minutes the fullness signal is not strong, then that's the time to eat something else, but if the fullness signal is saying, 'I've had enough', you can choose to move on with your day.

Choice 3: When you are eating, ask yourself, 'Do I have hunger?'

Initially, you might wonder, 'How will I know if I am full?' When looking for a signal that you have eaten enough, the answer is not to eat until you are uncomfortably full or even stuffed, but instead to use the same test that French people do. France's cuisine is world renowned, yet the French do not have the same problem with weight that we do in the UK. In French, when someone is hungry they say, '*J'ai faim*', which literally translated means, 'I *have* hunger.' When they finish eating they say, '*Je n'ai pas faim*', which means, 'I *don't have* hunger.' This is a very good approach for judging if you have eaten enough. Choose to pause frequently during a meal and ask yourself, 'If I had hunger at the start of eating, do I have hunger now?' If you conclude, '*Je n'ai pas faim*, I don't have hunger', then stop eating at that point. This approach will guide you to eat when you are hungry and to stop when the hunger is no longer there.

Choice 4: Choose to avoid eating foods that are 'Hunger in a Packet'

When you eat foods that your body quickly breaks down into sugar, insulin sweeps that sugar into fat storage before your body has had a chance to use it. The rapid lock-up into storage of the fuel you have just eaten explains why, very soon after eating these foods, you will be hungry again. This biology means we can reframe foods like sandwiches, breakfast cereal, pasta, biscuits, cakes and pastries – as Hunger in a Packet. The next time you see these foods, remind yourself that there's no point eating them because you will be just as hungry afterwards. Hunger in a Packet does not make you feel full.

Choice 5: Eat food, not calories

When you eat Programme foods you will tap back into your hunger and fullness hormone messages. This means that your body will naturally regulate the amount that you eat, just as it was designed to do. You will eat when you are hungry and stop when you are full and you will not need to think about the word 'calorie' ever again. Like many of my patients, you might have an encyclopaedic knowledge of the calorie content of hundreds of foods. I am delighted to tell my patients, and you too, that this knowledge is of no further use to you and you can now free up that precious brain space for other far more important and useful information.

By listening to your hunger and fullness signals there is no need to count, weigh or measure food. Food is here to nourish your mind and body and to be enjoyed. When you eat food in the same way your grandparents did, no equipment, notebook, app or calculator is required. Instead, all you need is the messaging system between your gut and your brain that has guided human eating for millennia.

CHAPTER 3

The Eating Window

**'The Eating Window sets you free and it puts
you in control because it's your decision to
set the times that work for you. I eat between
specific times and then I don't think about
food. It really gives you a life away from food.'**
Marcia, lost 5 stone (32kg)

If your parents or grandparents ever said to you, 'No eating
between meals', or 'Don't go to bed on a full stomach', or
even, 'The kitchen is closed!' then, although they probably
didn't know it at the time, their food wisdom about when to
eat and when not to eat was tapping into the powerful health
advantages of the Eating Window.

The Eating Window allows you to use the science behind
the statement: *When* you eat is as important as *what* you eat.
The idea is to choose to eat at specific times and to choose
other periods when you don't eat. By doing this you will be
changing the way your body's hormones and genes work,
using your biology to boost your health and drive your weight
loss.

Insulin – your all-day eating companion

From the moment that we wake up until the time we go to bed, the day presents an almost endless stream of eating opportunities. Breakfast, then a morning coffee break before lunch, followed by a mid-afternoon top-up. A little something when we get home, then dinner and perhaps some late-evening snacking.

If you wake up at 7am and go to bed at 11pm, that's sixteen hours of almost continual eating. And every time you eat, even if you are eating Programme foods, some sugar will end up in your blood. This means that insulin (the fat controller) will be constantly sweeping your continuous fuel intake into fat storage.

The Eating Window will free you from the company of the fat controller and its all-day sweeping. Instead, when you use an Eating Window, insulin levels will run low and you will stop fat storing.

Choosing to sweep or choosing to unlock

If you want to tap into the weight-loss advantage of the Eating Window, you can divide your day into two time periods. The first is a period when you can choose to eat if you are hungry. During this time, we say that your Eating Window is open. When you open your Eating Window and eat your first food of the day, there will be a small increase in the amount of sugar in your blood and insulin will arrive with its broom and start sweeping into storage.

After your last eating opportunity of the day, we say that your Eating Window closes. By closing your Eating Window, you have decided that, for this period of time, you will not be eating any food. With no food coming into your body, insulin is not needed to sweep sugar out of the blood.

When insulin levels are low, the fat controller puts down its broom and instead picks up its bunch of keys. These keys (low insulin levels) unlock stored body fat, which can now be broken down and released from fat storage. The result of this is you lose weight.

The aim of the Eating Window is to minimize the amount of time that high insulin levels are sweeping into fat storage (when your Eating Window is open) and to maximize the amount of time that low insulin (when your Eating Window is closed) is unlocking your fat and you lose weight.

A state-of-the-art, self-fuelling machine

At the start of the chapter, my patient Marcia shared with us, 'I eat between specific times and then I don't think about food.' What Marcia is so beautifully describing is the liberation of not feeling hungry when her Eating Window is closed. This happens because the body is a brilliant state-of-the-art, self-fuelling machine.

Your body has energy stored in three fuel tanks: your liver, your muscles and your body fat. When you close your Eating Window and you stop eating, rather than running on food, your body instead gets its energy by tapping into these fuel tanks. After a few hours, the stored fuel in your liver and muscles will be used up. It is then that you can tap into your third fuel tank: body fat.

When your Eating Window is closed, by using its stored energy, your body can fuel itself, without the need for you to eat anything. This is exactly what it is designed to do. We have these fuel tanks in anticipation of being able to call on them daily to use their stored energy when we need to.

If instead, we eat from breakfast right through to bedtime, we never give the body a chance to tap into its main fuel tank – body fat. Rather than being called upon regularly to release its stored fuel, instead body fat becomes a larger and larger – yet redundant – energy store, which we carry with us in the form of excess weight.

An Eating Window is not the same as a low-calorie diet

Choosing not to eat when your Eating Window is closed is very different from restricting your food intake on a low-calorie diet. These diets usually advise 'eating little and often' while basing food choices on low-fat carbohydrates, like diet crackers, breakfast cereal and low-calorie ready meals. This way of eating keeps insulin levels high, preventing you from tapping into the stored energy in your fuel tanks. With the body's energy stores locked up and not enough food coming in, the starvation response that we looked at in Chapter 2 is activated.

In contrast, by using an Eating Window, you are not under-fuelling your body. You are simply keeping your eating within a defined period of time. What's more, when your Eating Window is closed and insulin levels run low, all your energy needs are still being met because your body will use the energy in your fuel stores to run off.

Breakfast at sunrise

Insulin is not the only hormone that sends messages to your body's fuel tanks. Other hormones, including glucagon, instruct your body's fuel tanks to release some of their stored energy just before you wake up. This early morning tapping into your fuel tanks powers you up for the start of the day. You can think of this as your hormones serving up breakfast at sunrise, using fuel that you had stored exactly for this purpose. If you then wake up and eat straight away, you will be eating a 'second' breakfast before the day has really begun.

Insulin is also the disease controller

Like all hormones, insulin is meant to run at a precise, perfectly calibrated level within your body. When you have too much or too little of any hormone you will become unwell, and this is also true of insulin.

In today's world, it is possible to run insulin levels far in excess of those of past generations and much higher than the body needs. High insulin levels are a consequence of food choices as well as eating continuously through the day and, as we'll see in later chapters, not exercising and being sleep deprived. Over time, high insulin levels damage the body, contributing to the development of illnesses such as high blood pressure, heart disease and certain cancers (through insulin's stimulation of cell growth).

So insulin is the fat controller, and it is also the 'disease controller'. The good news is that you can choose to reduce insulin levels through what you eat and *when* you eat. If you choose to have a period of time when your Eating Window is closed, insulin levels will run low and you will be shutting out the disease controller.

Using your Eating Window to keep your body healthy and strong

Closing your Eating Window gives your body a period of time to do something else aside from eating, digesting and metabolizing food. This is very important. Today, we can easily fall into the habit of continually eating, snacking and grazing, but the human body was simply not designed to deal with constantly incoming food.

For most of human evolution, food was difficult to come by and was hard-won. Our ancestors would naturally have closed their Eating Window for many hours – or even days – usually because food was unavailable.

This break from having to digest and metabolize incoming food gives the body an opportunity to carry out other essential functions, such as reducing levels of inflammation, making new brain connections and repairing and maintaining the body. These processes are controlled by your genes, which can be 'switched on' or 'switched off' depending on whether you are eating (Eating Window open) or not eating (Eating Window closed).

When your Eating Window is closed, inflammation levels in your body will fall. While inflammation plays a powerful part in your body's response to injury or infection, factors such as stress, sleep deprivation and lack of exercise can cause constantly high levels of inflammation. Continuous, unchecked inflammation is associated with conditions like heart disease, cancer, dementia and depression. Closing your Eating Window influences your inflammation genes (such as the SIRT genes), resulting in dialled-down inflammation and a reduced risk of developing these illnesses.

A closed Eating Window also affects the genes in your brain (such as the BDNF gene) that activate a process called neuro-plasticity. Neuroplasticity describes how your brain remodels and reorganizes itself, including making new connections between your brain cells. Your brain's ability to change and restructure itself is essential for learning new skills and maintaining brain health as we age.

One last important gene to mention is the mTOR gene. When you close your Eating Window, the mTOR gene is switched off and your body's repair processes begin. Old, damaged cell parts are repaired or removed and new, healthy cell machinery develops. These vital repair and regeneration processes are known collectively as autophagy. Autophagy is so meaningful for good physical and mental health that Yoshinori Ohsumi, the scientist who pioneered this field, was awarded the Nobel Prize in Medicine in 2016 for his ground-breaking autophagy research.

So you can see that if your body is always eating, digesting and metabolizing food because your Eating Window never closes, these vital restorative processes cannot take place. However, if instead you choose to close your Eating Window for a set period of time every day, you will be giving your body the time it needs to repair, reset and regenerate, allowing you to become an even stronger and healthier version of yourself.

Important reasons to close your Eating Window include:

1. Running low insulin levels, which will lead to fat breakdown and weight loss as well as reducing your risk for insulin-driven diseases.
2. Giving your body the time to carry out essential repairs and resets.

CHOICES

Choice 1: Define your Eating Window timings

If you are choosing to tap into the weight-loss and health advantages of the Eating Window, the first thing to do is to decide on your timings along the line of these four statements:

1. My Eating Window opens at . . . o'clock. This is the time of day that I choose to first eat something.
2. My Eating Window is open for . . . hours. During this period of time I can choose to eat if I am hungry.
3. My Eating Window closes at . . . o'clock. This is the time that I choose to stop eating for the rest of the day.
4. My Eating Window is closed for . . . hours. During this period of time I am choosing not to eat.

I always ask my patients to choose their own timings because only they know what works for them. When you are deciding on the timings that suit you, it's useful to consider the question, 'When do I first feel hungry?' Most people are not hungry first thing in the morning, but they might be in the habit of eating when they wake up because they have been told that, 'Breakfast is the most important meal of the day.'

As we discussed in Chapter 2, your gut will send out a ghrelin hunger hormone text message when it requires you to eat something. If you are not hungry first thing in the morning, your ghrelin message is not strong because your body does not need or want food at that time. This may be because your hormones have already tapped into your fuel stores (see page 53) just before you have woken up, so your body is now powered up for the next few hours without the need for you to eat anything else.

The key here is to listen to your body. Then, when your ghrelin hunger message first feels strong, that is the time to open your Eating Window. Many of my patients tell me this happens sometime between about 11am and 2pm.

If we take a time somewhere in the middle, then statement 1 would read:

1. My Eating Window opens at 12pm (midday). This is when I choose to first eat something.

It is up to you to decide how long your Eating Window is open for. As well as thinking about when you tend to feel hungry, it's also helpful to take into account your schedule and household routine.

When you are looking at a typical day, it might be that eating dinner at 7.30pm works for you and after this, at 8pm, you close your Eating Window.

This means that statements 2, 3 and 4 would read:

2. My Eating Window is open for eight hours (12pm midday to 8pm). During this period of time I can choose to eat if I am hungry.
3. My Eating Window closes at 8pm. This is the time that I choose to stop eating for the rest of the day.
4. My Eating Window is closed for sixteen hours (8pm to 12pm midday the following day). During this period of time I am choosing not to eat.

When my patients work out their answers to statements 1 to 4, the majority will decide on an Eating Window that is open for eight hours and closed for sixteen hours, a duration that the science tells us will result in many health and weight loss benefits. One of the things that works well about this eight-hours-open, sixteen-hours-closed approach is that, since up to half of window closure time is spent asleep, you will be fat burning from the comfort of your own duvet.

Choice 2: Don't go to bed on a full stomach

Speaking of sleep, there is great wisdom in the adage, 'Don't go to bed on a full stomach.' Going to bed immediately after eating will set you up for issues such as heartburn, acid reflux and disrupted sleep because the sleeping human body is not well adapted to having a large amount of food in its gut.

Additionally, when you eat right up until bedtime, it will take time for insulin levels to fall. This means that instead of capitalizing on sleep time as 'easy-win' hours for fat burning (low insulin/keys out unlocking), you will instead waste some of these hours because you will have gone to bed while insulin is still sweeping.

In practice, the 'Don't go to bed on a full stomach' wisdom means choosing to close your Eating Window at least two hours before you go to bed, so that, when defining your timings, your fifth statement would read:

5. I choose to close my Eating Window at least two hours before I go to bed.

Choice 3: Use additional Eating Window know-how

There is some more great know-how to help you to easily use and enjoy the Eating Window.

First, if you like to drink tea or coffee in the morning, either black or with a small amount of milk, then you can continue to do this while your Eating Window still remains closed. If you are being technically correct, the caffeine and lactose (natural milk sugar) will cause a small increase in the amount of sugar and insulin in your blood, but not enough to impact on the weight-loss benefits of your Eating Window.

Many of my patients don't want to eat in the morning but would find it difficult not to drink tea or coffee. What I advise them is, 'Don't let the perfect be the enemy of the good.' If your morning cup of tea or coffee allows you to easily keep your Eating Window closed until late morning or early afternoon, then go for it!

Second, and on the same theme, when your Eating Window is closed, you are only choosing not to eat food. You can still drink water and hot drinks like coffee and tea, as described above, as well as herbal or fruit teas.

The third tip is to look carefully at the wording of Statement 2:

2. My Eating Window is open for . . . hours. During this period of time I can choose to eat if I am hungry.

You'll notice that the second sentence says, 'I can choose to eat *if* I am hungry', which means that you aren't trying to eat as much as possible while your Eating Window is open. Instead, you are choosing to eat when your hunger hormone signal is strong. In practice, most of my patients tell me that by tuning into their hunger–fullness messages, they end up eating about twice a day; once when they first open their Eating Window and again in the evening at dinner time, and they might have a snack in between.

Lastly, while your Eating Window is open, you can sometimes choose to have a 'micro-closure'. A micro-closure is the hours when you choose not to eat while your Eating Window is open. So if you finish your first meal of the day at 12.30pm and then have dinner at 6.30pm, in between you will have a six-hour micro-closure, which will allow insulin levels to fall.

There is no right or wrong approach to micro-closures – remember, if your hunger signal is strong between meals, then listen to your body's needs and eat something. Rather, a micro-closure is for the days when you aren't hungry between meals. At these times, you can choose not to eat a snack, allowing insulin to stop sweeping and to instead move into unlocking mode.

Choice 4: Choose thoughtful evening eating

One of the big advantages of closing your Eating Window at a particular time in the evening is that it breaks the habit of eating just for the sake of it. For example, you might be in the habit of snacking after dinner even though your hunger hormone message is not strong.

If you find yourself cruising the kitchen after dinner and

saying to yourself, 'I could eat some cheese, but I shouldn't, well, just a bit . . .' you will discover that telling yourself, 'I am choosing not to eat right now, my Eating Window is closed', makes your decision clear, freeing you from this internal back-and-forth chatter.

It tends to be easier to avoid snacking late in the evening when you reassure yourself that this food will still be available to you in the morning, and if you want to eat it when you wake up, of course you can. 'I'll eat it in the morning', is a powerful phrase because it stops your mind panicking and thinking, 'I must have it now.' Usually when you wake up in the morning, a combination of the sunrise hormone-energy boost and your mind being on other things means the urge to eat these foods will have disappeared.

Instead, this will now be a new day. Your Eating Window will be up and running once again and you will be using the brilliance of your body's biology to power you towards good health and weight-loss success.

CHAPTER 4

Gut bacteria

'I went to see Saira and joined her group
because I had a hope – the hope that she knew
a secret and might have a magic wand and I
would become slim and healthy. I was almost
right! She didn't have a magic wand, but she
knew the *secret*. She called that secret *science*.'
Gabriella, lost 3 stone 11lb (24kg)

Over one hundred trillion bacteria live in your gut. If this
sounds like a large number, it is – you contain more bacteria
cells than you do human cells and there are many more bacteria genes in your body than human genes. Taken together,
this makes you more bacteria than human being.

Your gut bacteria are not simply passive passengers, instead
they support essential functions within your body, which we
humans are unable to carry out without their help. What your
gut bacteria get in return for their work is food. The food you
eat feeds your gut bacteria too, which means that every time
you eat, you are in fact 'eating for two'.

Your gut bacteria are like workers on a factory production

line, which turn the food you eat into output products. These gut bacteria products profoundly affect your health, including your appetite and your weight. If you eat in a way that nourishes your gut bacteria, then you will be supporting them to make output products that control your weight and keep you feeling full.

Your gut bacteria factory – ramping up your appetite-control production line

The output of your gut bacteria factory depends on the foods that you put into the production line. When you eat certain foods, such as fibre and protein, your gut bacteria whir away to make a range of appetite-suppressing substances.

Fibre is a form of carbohydrate found in plant-based foods. You cannot digest fibre but your gut bacteria can. So when you eat fibre it is your gut bacteria (not you) that digest and ferment it. The end products of this gut bacteria–fibre production line are substances called short-chain fatty acids, which have a wide range of functions in your body – including suppressing your appetite. These gut bacteria appetite suppressants make you feel full by increasing the strength of the fullness hormone text messages between your gut and your brain. And short-chain fatty acids also work directly in your brain, where they turn up the fullness dial in its appetite control centre (the hypothalamus).

Your gut bacteria can also suppress your appetite when you feed them protein. Amazingly, the substance produced by your gut bacteria in response to the protein you eat is almost identical to a brain chemical that is your body's most potent appetite suppressant.

Your Programme foods, such as fibre and protein, have been carefully chosen to feed you and to feed your gut bacteria. Eating in this way supports your gut bacteria to make products that control your eating, allowing you to effortlessly end a meal. This has nothing to do with 'willpower' or having a 'good day' and everything to do with running a busy bacteria factory deep in your gut that is working hard every day to keep you feeling full.

'Diversity is our strength'

If your gut bacteria workers had a motto, it would be: 'Diversity is our strength.' This is because a diverse gut bacteria workforce has the skill set to produce a range of different products that help to control your weight and keep you healthy.

Eating today's standard low-fibre, low-protein, high-sugar, ultra-processed diet supplies the same limited foods to your gut bacteria again and again. With a restricted number of parts to work with, you will end up recruiting more of one type of gut bacteria to run the busy production lines, while losing the bacteria that have little to do. After a while, you will lose diversity in your gut bacteria workforce.

The hallmark of an unhealthy gut bacteria is where one type of bacteria dominates and other types are either present in low numbers or have disappeared altogether. This is a pattern seen in people carrying extra weight and is so well established that by analysing your stool (poo), it is possible for scientists to predict, without ever having met you, whether you are likely to be overweight.

If you are overweight, then you too might have developed this particular gut bacteria composition. What this means for your everyday weight control is that your gut bacteria are extra efficient at extracting energy from your food, releasing more calories than a lean person's gut bacteria, even if you are both eating in exactly the same way. (This is yet another reason why calorie counting is unhelpful – the calories on a food label tell us nothing about how many calories your own composition of gut bacteria will release from that food.)

If you think your gut bacteria might fit this pro-weight gain profile, don't worry. There is lots of practical advice coming up about how to put this right. In fact, the science tells us we can transform the gut bacteria within days when we change the way we feed it.

A body weight transplant

Even more evidence for the influence of the gut bacteria on weight comes from a game-changing experiment. In this research, scientists extracted gut bacteria from the faeces (poo) of obese laboratory mice and transplanted the obese mice's gut bacteria into normal-weight mice. After the gut bacteria

---

transplant, an extraordinary thing happened. The lean mice, without any change in their diet, became obese too. They now had gut bacteria inside them working to make them overweight.

You might be wondering if the same applies to humans – can weight be transferred from person to person? Faecal microbiota transplantation is an emerging therapy that transplants gut bacteria from a healthy person (the donor) into the gut of a person who is unwell (the recipient). The premise is that the healthy bacteria from the donor will produce health-giving substances in the gut of the unwell recipient. However, it was when a woman who received a gut bacteria transplant from her overweight daughter experienced a 2 stone 5lb (15kg) weight gain that this first suggested gut bacteria can transmit body weight between humans. Experts now recommend that gut bacteria donors should be a healthy weight.

When we discuss this story in our group sessions, my patients often follow up with a clever question: if the gut bacteria from an overweight person can transmit weight gain, could a gut bacteria transplant from a lean person help others to lose weight? Science and medicine are always moving forward, so in the future, perhaps a gut bacteria transplant will become a weight-loss treatment. However, once my patients have heard the practical advice you'll now read about, they conclude, why receive someone else's gut bacteria when we already have one hundred trillion of our own, which will work to keep us lean and healthy if we feed them right?

CHOICES

Choice 1: Eat plenty of fibre every day

One of the reasons the Programme is so effective is that my patients don't feel hungry. By eating plenty of fibre-rich Programme foods, like vegetables, fruits, nuts, seeds and lentils, my patients have harnessed the power of their gut bacteria to produce appetite-suppressing substances that leave them with a feeling of contented fullness after eating.

Fibre increases the diversity of your gut bacteria, changing them from the composition of a person carrying more weight to that of a lean individual, with a workforce that is less efficient at extracting calories from the food you eat.

And fibre also has a further weight control advantage – by holding in the natural sugars found in foods like fruits and vegetables, fibre makes it harder for your body to release the food's sugar. So high-fibre foods keep the after-meal rise in your blood sugar levels slow and controlled, resulting in less insulin sweeping and less fat storage (see pages 9–10).

Good sources of fibre

By choosing to eat at least 30g of fibre a day, you will enjoy all of its health benefits. As you know, the Programme is not about weighing, measuring or counting food; but to get your eye in, it's a good idea to keep a check on how much fibre you're eating.

Vegetables are the best way to get fibre into your diet – a 200g serving of Brussels sprouts or cabbage both contain a robust 10g of fibre.

Seeds are another good source of fibre. For example, eating 2 tablespoons of flaxseed (linseed) – which contains 9g of fibre – straight off the spoon every day, washed down with a large glass of water, will be good for your gut bacteria and will also keep you regular.

Lentils, beans (not baked beans, which are high in sugar) and chickpeas are a good source of a substance related to fibre called resistant starch, which your gut bacteria factory is also adept at working with.

Choice 2: Eat your vegetables!

Vegetables nourish you and they nourish your gut bacteria, which puts them at the centre of your Programme eating. The joy of vegetables is their abundance of goodness, including fibre, vitamins, minerals and phytonutrients.

If you aren't keen on vegetables, then you'll be amazed at how the Programme transforms you into a 'natural' vegetable eater. This will happen because eating vegetables on the Programme tastes good. Take a look at the recipes on pages 219–89 for lots of ideas that will give you a new appreciation for all the varied vegetable tastes and flavours available to you. Soon you will develop a trusted repertoire, like adding butter to your steamed broccoli, drizzling olive oil on a rocket and walnut salad or baking mushrooms with some herbs and feta cheese. These are just three examples of the hundreds of ways by which, done the Programme way, vegetables can be given the chance to shine as the delicious, health-boosting foods they are.

Eating a rainbow

Phytonutrients are a diverse group of naturally occurring plant substances that your gut bacteria use to make numerous products that powerfully improve your health. Many phytonutrient-rich foods come in bright, beautiful colours – sunshine yellow turmeric, for example, or the deep mauve of an aubergine. By eating these foods, you are 'eating a rainbow' and embracing foods that nature blessed with this dazzling kaleidoscope, while turning away from foods that are only colourful because an E number was added to them.

At the start of this chapter my patient Gabriella described how her weight issue had finally been answered by 'knowing the secret' – the science she had learnt in the Programme. Science improves our health when we apply it in a practical way to our everyday lives, an idea that is at the heart of the Programme. I hope this chapter has shown how you can use this new and exciting gut bacteria science to change the foods you eat – and rather than eating for one, you will now start eating for two (or, to be precise, one hundred trillion). When you do this, within just a few days your gut bacteria will change, quickly transforming from a workforce that was not helping with your weight control into a rebuilt, reinvigorated dream team that works every day to keep you lean.

CHAPTER 5

Movement

'Before I started this programme, I was a
mess, emotionally and physically. I can't
thank you enough for changing my life. For
setting me free. For empowering me with
the science on how my body works. Now,
after so many years of being trapped in a
rotten cocoon, I feel like a beautiful butterfly,
free and happy! And it's all due to this life-
changing programme. A million thank yous!'
Farah, lost 2 stone (13kg)

Human beings were designed to move. Put another way,
being still too much of the time is not good for us. If the
word 'exercise' doesn't currently fill you with pleasure, this
chapter will help to change that. By understanding the science of movement, you will be able to discard the old way of
thinking of exercise as a way to 'burn off calories'. Instead,
you will see that exercise plays a powerful role in keeping
insulin levels running low, which is the link between exercise
and weight loss.

Exercise is a potent prescription so it comes with side-effects. But unlike those related to medication, the side-effects of exercise feel good, including reduced blood pressure, stable blood sugar levels, strong muscles, an efficient heart, a bright mood and good-quality sleep.

Once you know about all the weight-loss and health advantages of exercise, this chapter will be your guide to finding a way of moving every day that is right for you, that feels good and that will propel you into a future that is full of good health.

Why 'burning it off' doesn't work

Before we look at how exercise helps you to lose weight, let's get out of the 'burning it off' mindset. This is part of the 'calories-in-calories-out' way of thinking, which is sometimes used to offset certain food choices, like eating biscuits because, 'I'm going to the gym later.'

The problem here is that the biscuits affect the body over and above weight gain. Aside from the harmful effects of ultra-processed foods on the gut bacteria (Chapter 4) and on the rest of the body (Chapters 1, 2, 7, 8 and 13), the sugar itself in the biscuits causes damage.

Although most of the sugar will be swept into your three fuel tanks (your liver, muscles and body fat), some will be deposited in other parts of your body, including your heart, your kidneys and your brain. In time, these delicate body parts become 'sugar-coated' (a process known as glycation). Glycation causes problems such as heart disease and declining kidney function, and studies now suggest a link between overloading the brain with sugar and dementia. So you can see that going to the gym to compensate for food choices can't undo the damage that these foods do. It's not possible to outrun a bad diet.

'Burning it off' also supposes that you can immediately use up the energy from the biscuits as soon as you hit the gym. In fact, you need to work through each of the body's fuel tanks in turn. First, the energy stored in your muscles (300 calories-worth) will be used, then your liver fuel (1,000 calories). Once you have used up this stored energy, you will then start to use your third fuel tank, body fat, where most of the excess sugar from the biscuits has ended up. But getting through the first 1,300 calories could mean exercising for a few hours, which isn't realistic for most of us.

As you can see, most of the exercise that we have time to do – say, forty minutes of gardening or swimming for half an hour – will be powered by the body's muscle and liver fuel tanks, while fat stores remain undented. I hope that knowing this will free you from the inaccurate link between exercise and 'burning it off'.

What's the point in exercising then?

In normal biology, insulin should be able to easily sweep excess sugar out of the blood and into the liver without encountering any resistance to its sweeping. The liver can deal with a bit of sugar, storing some as fuel and converting any extra into fat, which is sent to body fat for storage (resulting in weight gain).

A problem arises when we eat a lot of foods like breakfast cereal, bread, biscuits, fruit juice and fizzy drinks, which overload the liver with sugar. The liver is now forced to convert more and more sugar into fat, which gets stuck in the liver, causing unhealthy congestion – a condition known as fatty liver. To protect itself, the liver shuts the door on insulin, making it difficult for insulin to sweep in any more sugar. This is known as insulin resistance and is the root cause of chronic metabolic illnesses like weight gain, high blood pressure, type 2 diabetes and polycystic ovarian syndrome.

Insulin does not like to be met with a closed door, so it tries to overcome the lock-out (resistance) by recruiting more insulin janitors. The result is continuously high insulin levels trying to break down the door (overcome the insulin resistance).

These high insulin levels drive weight gain because body fat is the one fuel tank that has an unlimited storage capacity and never closes its door on insulin.

You can see that a vicious cycle has developed. Eating a high-sugar diet leads to insulin resistance. Insulin resistance leads to high insulin levels. High insulin levels promote fat storage and weight gain. Weight gain increases levels of inflammation in the body, which drives even more insulin resistance.

You might think this is all biologically fascinating, but isn't this chapter supposed to be about exercise? Well, guess what exercise does – exercise reduces insulin resistance, breaking you free from this vicious cycle.

When you exercise, your muscles pull in sugar from your blood without needing insulin to sweep it in. As a result, the amount of sugar in your blood falls. The back-up janitors that had been called in can now be stood down. Insulin levels fall and you lose weight. When you lose weight, inflammation levels in the body decrease and insulin resistance reduces further.

The link between exercise and weight loss is the melting away of insulin resistance. Along with choosing low-sugar foods and having an Eating Window, exercise supports you to reduce your insulin levels. So you can see that the Programme is not a 'low-carb plan' – it is a low-insulin way of life.

Type 2 diabetes and insulin resistance

The cause of type 2 diabetes is not high blood sugar. This is a common misperception because so much of the treatment focuses on controlling blood sugar levels using tablets and injections. In fact, high blood sugar is a *symptom* of type 2 diabetes, while the *cause* of this condition is insulin resistance.

At a certain tipping point, no matter how much insulin is produced, there is too much resistance to overcome and insulin can't sweep enough sugar out of the blood. Blood sugar levels start to run high and type 2 diabetes is diagnosed. Whereas medication will treat the high blood-sugar symptom, reducing insulin resistance through lifestyle choices, like exercise, targets the root cause of type 2 diabetes.

Exercise and good physical health

Exercise has physical health benefits for two reasons. First, the mechanical aspect of exercise – calling on your heart to pump, your lungs to breathe and your muscles to contract – makes your body stronger. Second, by reducing insulin resistance, insulin levels in the body run lower. Illnesses that are driven by insulin resistance, such as high blood pressure, fatty liver and polycystic ovarian syndrome, improve. And once insulin can sweep sugar out of the blood without encountering resistance, blood sugar levels fall to normal levels, reversing type 2 diabetes, which is a common Programme outcome.

Exercise and good mental health

If you exercise regularly you will enjoy considerable mental health benefits too. When you exercise, feel-good brain chemicals called endorphins lift your mood, lower stress, reduce anxiety and give you that after-exercise 'buzz'. To understand the power of the exercise-endorphin effect, let's break down the name: 'endo' meaning internal or within the body, and 'orphin' from the word morphine, a strong opiate painkiller drug. Put another way, endorphins are our 'internal morphine'. Except, of course, no medication is needed, and there is no risk of side-effects. To tap into those potent feel-good endorphins, you just need to keep your body moving.

Exercise will also improve the quality of your sleep. By

moving your body during the day, you will have a healthy sense of tiredness at night, as well as a mental calm that makes it easier to fall asleep.

And as your body becomes stronger and fitter, this will also do wonders for your confidence and self-esteem. A body that is being used to its full potential is a body that feels good to live in.

This is how my patient Farah felt, whose words start this chapter. She describes emerging from a 'rotten cocoon' and then taking flight 'like a beautiful butterfly, free and happy!' By exercising, she was now flying through the day.

If the idea of flying through the day currently seems very far off, the upcoming practical advice will support you to build exercise into your day. These Programme choices will guide you away from being still and towards embracing movement as an invigorating and enjoyable way of life.

CHOICES

Choice 1: Getting started – make a plan

If you aren't sure how to get started with exercise, the first thing to do is to make a plan. Your exercise is far more likely to happen when you block out a period of time in your diary, in the same way that you would book in a meeting or social commitment. This forward planning will also dispel any idea you might have that you don't have time to exercise. Even my busiest patients, some with more than one job as well as family commitments, found that when they looked at their schedule, they were able to carve out time to exercise once they decided that it was important to them.

How long you exercise for depends on your current level of fitness. Please don't worry if at first you aren't exercising for long and think that this somehow doesn't count – it does! If you go from no exercise to ten minutes, that's ten minutes more than you were doing before. The brilliance of the human body is that the more you use it, the better it works. So as you continue to get out there and keep on moving, your strength and stamina will increase and your ability to exercise will naturally build up.

Choice 2: Enjoy it!

If you think back to when you were a child, you didn't exercise to melt away insulin resistance. You played football or ran around the playground because you enjoyed it. The same is true as an adult. Choose exercise that gives you pleasure and it is more likely that you will keep on doing it.

We tend to enjoy things we are suited to. If you compare a rugby player with a marathon runner, they have very different physiques, yet both are elite athletes. In the same way, certain types of exercise will particularly suit your own build and constitution. There is no right exercise, only exercise that is right for you.

It's also time to move away from the idea that exercise has to hurt or feel uncomfortable to be working – the 1980s 'no pain no gain' philosophy has no place in the Programme.

Instead, when we do exercise that suits us and that we enjoy, exercise feels good.

You might decide to play a team sport with your friends, do lengths at your local pool, go to the gym or cycle to work. Or you might choose walking as your daily exercise. If so, you can monitor your activity by counting your steps on your phone or fitness tracker. Ten thousand steps a day tends to be a popular target. There is no scientific evidence to support this number, but it's one that many of my patients adopt because they find it doable, providing them with a wealth of physical and mental health benefits. Be kind to yourself – see how many steps you can do in the here and now, then encourage yourself to increase the number of steps as your fitness increases.

Choice 3: Choose to make the world your gym

Often exercise is seen as being an hour at the gym or forty lengths of the pool. While these are great activities, exercise is not an isolated event that can be done and then ticked off until tomorrow. Exercise is movement and movement is an all-day, every day, event. You'll be amazed at all the opportunities that daily life gives you to move when you look for them. Examples include:

- Changing your commute from still time to activity time by cycling or walking for some or all of the journey.
- Taking the stairs instead of the lift or escalator.
- Getting off the bus a few stops early and walking the rest of the way.

- Doing the school run on foot rather than driving.
- Running around with the kids at the playground or park rather than sitting on a bench.

In these examples you are not 'doing' exercise, it's just that you are an active person who is constantly looking out for opportunities to make the world your gym.

Choice 4: Make exercise the easy option

You are more likely to exercise when to do so is the easy choice. Making some small changes will get you big results when it comes to your motivation to exercise. You could set things up like this:

- Taking your trainers to work so that it's comfortable to walk all or part of the way home.
- Exercising with a friend so that you keep your commitment to them even if you don't feel like exercising that day.
- Keeping it local – you are more likely to exercise if you choose a convenient nearby gym or park than if you have to travel a long distance to make it happen.
- Leaving home earlier so that you can walk some of the way, rather than making the whole journey on public transport.
- Having your equipment readily accessible. For example, making it easy to wheel your bicycle straight out of the front door, rather than having to retrieve

it from a shed or spare room. Keeping your mat and hand weights in the room where you stream your workout video.

- Using a comfortable bag or basket on wheels to make shopping on foot a more attractive option than taking the car.

Choice 5: It's NEAT to fidget

There is another form of movement that helps us break free from being still – non-exercise activity thermogenesis or NEAT for short (there's more about NEAT in Chapter 14). NEAT uses up energy outside of formal activities like sports or exercise on seemingly trivial activities such as playing with a pen or tapping your foot. Children have a natural tendency towards NEAT, which is why they can't sit still for long. This constant movement – NEAT – is an important reason why young children are not usually overweight.

As we get older, our bodies tend to move out of NEAT mode. We can, though, choose to rediscover our childlike tendency for NEAT, which the evidence shows is associated with maintaining a healthy weight. Ideas for incorporating neat little bits of NEAT into your day include:

- Standing on public transport even when there are seats available.
- Changing your posture regularly when sitting.
- Playing with your pen in a meeting.

- Walking around when on a phone call.
- Going over to speak to your kids rather than shouting across the room.
- Offering to fetch something that has been left in another part of the house.
- Jumping up to answer the doorbell rather than waiting for someone else to go.
- Using a basket at the supermarket rather than a trolley when doing a small food shop.

Wherever you are with exercise today, I am certain that you will be able to use the science and practical advice in this chapter to free yourself from the old idea of exercise being something you should do to burn calories. This will now allow you to see exercise as an enjoyable way to keep your insulin levels running low, which will drive weight loss and other physical health improvements. Your mood will feel good too – exercise is 'first aid' for the mind. I didn't use to cycle, but when I found it made my commute to the hospital quicker and that I had some of my best ideas on my bike, I kept on going. Even when the hospital offered staff car parking permits during the Covid-19 pandemic, I continued to cycle because if there was ever a time for mind first aid, that was it.

I hope you can now reframe the idea of exercise from being something that feels uncomfortable or that requires special clothes or equipment to simply being about taking every opportunity to move. Whether it's the joy of gardening, the satisfaction of walking up the escalator, the mental clarity of yoga or the tingle in your cheeks after a bracing walk, once your body is regularly active you will feel so good you will always want to keep on moving.

CHAPTER 6

Sleep

**'Thank you for all your support. I am in the
controlling seat of my life and no longer a
passenger. The Programme has changed
my entire life, not just my weight.'**
Salma, lost 2 stone 1lb (13kg)

Nobody knows exactly why we sleep, but the universal consensus is that it is important. Sleep is a behaviour that we share in common with mammals throughout the natural world as varied as lions, bats and dolphins. For sleep to have persisted across all mammals, without evolution disposing of it in some, suggests that it is fundamental to life.

You might already be aware that sleep is essential for your mental and physical health, but you may be less familiar with the influence that sleep has on your weight. If you don't get enough sleep, your body's hormone levels will change to give you a boost that keeps you going the next day – but this hormone jump-start will also drive hunger and weight gain.

This chapter will explain the science of why sleep is important to your appetite, weight control and overall good health, and it will also guide you through the practical steps you can take to restore and improve your sleep. Once you are getting enough sleep, you will be running hormone levels that help you to lose weight and feel good.

Sleep – the ultimate reset

When you sleep, your body recharges and resets. Damage done to the body during the day is healed. Your brain is, quite literally, deep-cleaned by the fluid that surrounds it. Memories and thoughts from the day are organized and filed; 'It will all seem better in the morning', really does have a scientific underpinning. What's more, each cell in your body contains an internal clock, operating on a 24-hour cycle that sets the rhythm and the timing of all of your body's processes. These internal clocks need to be perfectly synchronized with each other and with your brain's master clock (the suprachiasmatic nucleus) so that every part of your body does the right thing at the right time, in the right way. During the day, your body's clocks become slightly out of synch with one another. Sleep resynchronizes them so that the next day, after a good night's sleep, they are all telling the same time again and your mind and body function at peak performance.

Your cortisol back-up generator

When we don't get enough sleep, our cell clocks are not reset and instead will be out of synch with each other and with the brain's master clock. As a result, body processes happen at the wrong time, or don't happen at all, and this does not feel good. In time, this disruption to our internal timetable can cause health problems, including weight gain.

In a normal sleep pattern, sometime after midnight, your adrenal glands click into gear and begin to increase production of the hormone cortisol. After a full night's sleep, your body's cortisol levels will reach a peak just before you wake up, launching you out of rest-sleep mode and into energized daytime mode. After this, cortisol levels begin to fall and by the late afternoon are at a quarter of the early morning peak.

As well as this day-to-day biology, cortisol is one of the body's 'stress' hormones. In this role, cortisol has evolved to be called upon infrequently when your body is under unusual or exceptional stress, such as fighting an infection or undergoing surgery.

The body sees sleep deprivation as a stress because it has not been adequately recharged overnight, but still needs to get up, walk, talk and function the next day. So cortisol levels now ramp up in their role as a stress hormone to push us through. Rather than the normal pattern of a morning cortisol rise that then tapers off, cortisol will instead continue to run high all day, functioning as a back-up generator to keep us going.

The problem is that our cortisol stress response was not designed to be running high day after day if we are frequently not getting enough sleep. The cortisol stress response is a testament to the resilience of the body to keep on going, but running high cortisol levels has a side-effect – it makes us put on weight.

Steroids and weight gain

Cortisol is a steroid hormone that is produced by your body. One way to frame the relationship between high cortisol levels (caused by sleep deprivation) and weight gain is that, if you have ever taken steroid tablets for a condition like asthma or arthritis, it is likely that the steroid medication made you put on weight.

Cortisol causes weight gain because it makes the body resistant to insulin. This makes insulin levels shoot up to try to overcome the body's resistance to it. So even if you are eating on-Programme, using an Eating Window and exercising, if you are sleep deprived, insulin (the fat controller) will run high the next day and you will be in fat-storage mode.

Lack of sleep makes us hungry

After a poor night's sleep it can be more difficult to make healthy eating choices, making it easy for old habits to slip back in. This, combined with the food industry's marketing messages, can lead a tired mind to believe that a sugar hit will be the recharge it needs. In fact, that sugar will be a ticket back on to the blood sugar rollercoaster, making us feel exhausted with its all-day surging and crashing.

When we are sleep deprived, levels of ghrelin – the stomach's hunger hormone message – run higher than usual, making us feel particularly hungry and at risk of overeating. In one research study, after just one night of inadequate sleep, the group who had slept for four hours ate 22 per cent more food the next day compared to the group who had slept for eight hours. In a week of sleep deprivation, this overeating could result in an extra day and a half's worth of food; or put another way, an eight-and-a-half-day eating week.

Calming the sleep-deprivation hormone storm

This is the sleep-deprivation hormone storm: ghrelin, the hunger hormone, is driving a voracious appetite; cortisol, the stress hormone, is running high and increased levels of insulin tip us into fat-storage mode.

But don't worry, you can use the Programme to improve your sleep, which will calm the hormone storm and make your day feel brighter. Life can be messy, busy and unpredictable, so I can't guarantee the advice I'm going to give you is a silver bullet that will always give you a perfect night's sleep. Instead, these choices are a framework that will allow you to steadily make changes to improve your sleep enough to keep the day ahead storm-free, giving you a well-slept weight-loss advantage.

CHOICES

Choice 1: Have a look at whether you are getting enough sleep

A question that my patients frequently ask me is, 'How much sleep should I be getting?' The answer to this is that we are all unique and there is no magic number of hours that will be right for everyone. Instead, you will know whether you are getting enough sleep if you wake up in the morning energized, feeling good and full of get-up-and-go for the day ahead.

If you don't currently feel this way, if you hit the snooze button until the very last minute and you are tired during the day, then without the need for tests or sleep-tracking devices, you can confidently conclude that you aren't getting enough sleep and it is time for a sleep audit.

<u>Take your own sleep audit</u>

During our session on sleep, I ask my patients to complete the following statements:

I go to bed at . . . o'clock.

I wake up at . . . o'clock.

I get . . . hours of sleep a night.

I find getting out of bed in the morning:
easy/moderately difficult/very difficult

I would encourage you to complete these statements yourself. Often my patients are surprised at how little sleep they are getting and their audit results motivate them to change their sleep routines, often reporting back that they are now feeling refreshed in the morning with far more energy for the day ahead.

Choice 2: What's stopping you going to bed early enough?

If your sleep audit and the way you feel when you wake up are telling you that you aren't getting enough sleep, the next step is to look at your evening routine, which might be impacting your sleep.

This is why I ask my patients to complete these statements:

These are the things that stop me from going to bed earlier:

1. . . . .

2. . . . .

Here are the two answers that my patients most frequently share:

1. Screen use.
2. Delaying going to bed to carve out some 'Me Time'.

Let's look at each of these answers, as they might be stealing your sleep time too.

Screen use: If you use a screen at night when your body is moving into the rest-sleep part of your 24-hour circadian cycle, then light from the screen will confuse your body's timetable. The blue light emitted by the screen hits the back of your eyes, sending a message to your brain's master clock that says, 'It's the awake phase, time for daytime processes to happen, like alertness and activity.' Rather than moving into rest mode, the screen's light stimulates ongoing wakeful processes in your body, pushing your 24-hour cycle off schedule. Now, instead of feeling sleepy, your mind is buzzing and alert.

Aside from the effect on your body's circadian timekeeping, screen-based activities tend to be emotionally disruptive. In the lead-up to sleep, your restful (parasympathetic) nervous system should be winding you down. Instead, your sympathetic (fight or flight) nervous system can be overactivated by screen content – difficult emails, upsetting social media content or overwrought TV shows.

If you feel that screens are your barrier to an earlier bedtime, you could choose an evening cut-off time when you put your phone and devices away. It is telling that many people who work in the tech industry choose to do this because they know how disruptive screen use can be before sleep.

Initially, some of my patients are quite resistant to these suggestions. But when we talk it through, the majority conclude that high cortisol, insulin resistance, hunger, irritability and weight gain are too high a price to pay for pre-sleep screen use.

The other sleep barrier that my patients often share is, 'I want to extend the evening because otherwise I feel like I don't have any Me Time', meaning time to myself when I'm not working or taking care of things at home. You might recognize how a busy day followed by an evening 'second shift' of family and household tasks can push your opportunity for Me Time to late at night.

One way to address this is to make a choice about the time you want to go to bed – a time that you know will give you enough sleep so that you feel good and energetic the next day. Let's say you decide on a 10:30pm bedtime. If you then review your evening activities you might identify changes that will give you more time to yourself. Do you have to do the laundry or can it wait until the morning? Are the out-of-hours emails urgent or just run-of-the-mill matters that you can look at when you are back at work – remember, before the internet, work was usually done at work!

If you review your evening, like my patients do, it is likely that you too can find ways to take back some of your evening for earlier Me Time that doesn't overstep into your precious sleep time. In the same way that parents set a bedtime for their children, as adults we can show ourselves that same care by establishing an evening routine and bedtime that give us a good night's sleep.

Choice 3: Reclaim and improve your sleep

Preparing to go to sleep is not just about the immediate few minutes before we get into bed. Instead, we can reframe the lead-up to sleep as being an all-day event. This might sound a bit surprising, but as you'll see, in addition to things like screen use immediately before bed, the things you do during the day, like exercising and drinking coffee, will also affect your sleep. Here is my Programme guide for putting you in pole position for a good night's sleep:

1. **Prepare your sleep environment**

   If you have ever looked after a baby, you'll remember the care that you took with their sleep environment, keeping the room dark and quiet and at the right temperature. You can now choose to apply the same care to yourself.

   This involves making sure your bedroom is dark, eliminating light from things like a clock radio or gaps in the curtains. You could also use an eye sleep mask if it's hard to make the bedroom dark enough. If you need an overnight light source outside your room, a plug-in nightlight that emits a soft orange glow is less confusing to your body's timekeeping than the light from a standard light bulb. And keeping your bedroom at about 20°C is a good temperature because it supports your body's natural drop in temperature during sleep.

Weighted blankets

Weighted blankets have become a popular sleep aid. I can't provide you with a clinical trial showing the benefits of a weighted blanket, but many of my patients tell me how using one relaxes them and improves their sleep. The blanket's weight can be chosen according to comfort and your own body weight. The premise is that the weight of the blanket envelops, soothes and calms your body, a bit like swaddling a baby or being given a big warm hug.

---

2. **Review your caffeine use**

Caffeine is a powerful brain stimulant, which is why drinking it feels so good. Exactly how long it takes your body to completely eliminate caffeine from the system is down to your genes, but in some people it can take up to twelve hours. For example, if you have a cup of tea at 4pm that caffeine might still be stimulating your brain after midnight, making it hard to fall asleep. So it's a good idea to review how much coffee and tea (including green tea) you are consuming and when you are drinking it. Many of my patients (some of whom thought they had sleep problems) are amazed at the improvement in their sleep once they have a stop time for their caffeine use. Since we don't know how fast each of us clears caffeine, a practical approach we have used in the Programme is to stop drinking caffeine at around midday. After this, some of my patients instead like to switch to decaffeinated tea and coffee, herbal teas or hot water.

3. **Exercise during the day**
   A body that has been physically active during the day is a body that will sleep well at night. One of the many benefits of exercise is that it improves your sleep quality. Parents of young children know that without enough exercise, their kids won't go to bed well and the same is true for us grown-ups. Aside from physically tiring your body out, the release of feel-good endorphins when you exercise has a calming effect on your mood, even hours later when you are dropping off to sleep. The one caveat is not to exercise too close to bedtime. Hormones like adrenaline that are released during exercise can make you feel more alert – a good thing during the day but not for winding down before sleep.

4. **Stop using a screen a couple of hours before you want to go to sleep**

This will be extremely beneficial for your evening wind-down, reclaiming your Me Time and going to sleep at your chosen time. Screen use also applies to using your phone to check the time overnight because the light emitted from the screen will disrupt your body's internal timekeeping. Here, a traditional bedside clock might help. Many of my patients tell me this has an extra benefit – their phone (and a homescreen full of notifications) is no longer the first thing they look at when they wake up. Instead, they now engage with their phone once they are out of bed, on their terms and when they are ready.

5. **Speak to your doctor if you are still having problems falling or staying asleep**

Once you've tried out these suggestions, if you are still experiencing sleep difficulties, then it's a good idea to speak to your doctor.

Common patterns I see include difficulty falling asleep, staying asleep or waking up very early in the morning. This kind of sleep disturbance might be due to low mood or anxiety and your doctor will be able to advise on the best treatment options for you.

It's also a good idea to speak to your doctor if you need to drink alcohol or take sleeping tablets to help you sleep. Even though they are sedatives, the resulting sleep quality will be poor, and these substances can be addictive.

Sometimes sleep can be interrupted by a condition called sleep apnoea, which is caused by narrowing of the windpipe during sleep. This results in breathing difficulties, poor-quality sleep, low energy the next day and, if left untreated, can cause long-term health problems. Symptoms of sleep apnoea include snoring, partner concerns about overnight breathing or falling asleep during the day. If you think you might have sleep apnoea, your doctor will be able to advise on the best next steps.

Some of my patients have no difficulty falling asleep but then wake up overnight, for example, to use the bathroom. If you have symptoms that interrupt your sleep, again, it's a good idea to consult your doctor as treating the underlying condition will improve your sleep quality.

Implementing changes to your sleep routines will take commitment and perseverance. My patients tell me that. But they also tell me that by using these suggestions they have been able to improve their sleep and many feel that this has been key to their weight-loss success. My patient Salma, whose bold words open the chapter, sums up this can-do approach: 'I am in the controlling seat of my life and no longer a passenger.' By using the Programme's sleep guide, Salma found a port in the sleep-deprivation hormone storm. Not every night went perfectly, that's not real life, but just as Salma did, you too can make enough changes so that your health and your weight-loss goals benefit from the power of sleep – the body's ultimate magic fix.

CHAPTER 7

Genes

'You have genuinely changed my life. I used
to be so jealous of people who could say no
to chocolate or open a pack of biscuits and
not finish them all. And now I don't even
want that stuff in my home! Just before I
started the Programme, I remember hearing
a panellist on *Loose Women* say, "I only eat
when I am hungry." I thought to myself,
wow, I wish I was like her. And now I am!'
Mital, lost 4 stone 8lb (29kg)

If your weight is higher than you would like it to be despite
trying numerous diets, then you might have asked yourself the
question, 'Why me?' Many of my patients have asked themselves the same thing. What they mean by this is, 'Why did I
develop a weight issue, while other people remain lean?' If your
current beliefs steer you towards blaming yourself, I would like
to gently guide you away from this mindset and instead suggest
an alternative answer to the question, 'Why me?'

Your genes.

Weight is one of many characteristics that is inherited within families through the passing on of genes from one generation to the next. Studies show that up to 70 per cent of your weight is set by your genes, which is only slightly less than the influence of your genes on your height. We instinctively understand that height runs in families, just as we're familiar with the idea that your genes make your eyes and skin a certain colour. However, what you might be less familiar with is that, in addition to these obvious inherited characteristics, your genes also give instructions to your body about your weight.

This might not be the news you were hoping for. On first reflection, you might worry that if your weight is influenced by your genes, and your genes are as they are, then it will be impossible for you to lose weight.

In fact, the outlook is much brighter than you might imagine. As you will see in this chapter, by eating in a way that works *with* your genes, you will find that any tendency you may have towards overeating significantly improves. So this chapter is a good news story because no matter the genetic hand that you have been dealt, once you get to know yourself better and understand which foods are going to work with your genes, you can still live at a weight that is right for you.

You and your genes

You can think of your genes as being your body's instruction manual, and when it comes to your weight, your gene instruction manual influences how your brain responds to eating certain foods. Depending on your individual set of genes, there might be certain trigger foods that can drive overeating, resulting in weight gain. But remember, this chapter has a good news message because once you've identified the trigger foods that don't seem to work with your unique genetic makeup, you can choose, just as my patients have done, to minimize consumption of these foods – or even to avoid them altogether.

How your genes affect your weight

Your weight is not regulated by any one single gene. Instead, we are each dealt a particular genetic hand in which different versions of weight-control genes are possible. These gene variants mean that while you could have one version of a particular weight-control gene, your partner, neighbour or colleague could have another. Each version of a weight-control gene can either increase or decrease the risk for weight gain. Cumulatively, each of these weight-control genes will contribute in a small way to an overall predisposition to be a particular weight.

Scientists have found that there is one gene in particular, called fat mass and obesity related transcript (or FTO for short), that is most strongly associated with the risk of weight gain. There are different versions of the FTO gene and the one that you have will influence whether you are more likely or less likely to gain weight.

About 50 per cent of us have a version of the FTO gene that is associated with a 3lb (1.5kg) weight increase (compared to people who don't have this version). Those of us who have this version of FTO are 20 per cent more likely to become obese. A further 16 per cent of us have a version of FTO that is associated with being 6lb (3kg) heavier. If we have this version, we are 50 per cent more likely to become obese. We will refer to this version of the FTO gene as FTO Risk.

Precisely how the FTO gene affects our weight is the subject of ongoing research. Evidence suggests that FTO influences food choices, and studies have shown that people with FTO Risk have a greater preference for, and might even overeat, sugary junk food compared to people who do not have the FTO Risk gene.

If you have the FTO Risk gene, and let's say you are at a buffet lunch where a huge array of food is available, you might be more likely than other people to choose ultra-processed, high-sugar foods like biscuits and pastries. Moreover, when other guests have put down their plates, you might be fighting the urge to return to the buffet table for another helping. If you have FTO Risk, the genetic hand you have been dealt might make it very hard, maybe even impossible, to stop once you start eating these sorts of foods. The advertisers instinctively knew who they were targeting when they told us, 'Once you pop, you can't stop.'

Why just one is never enough

In your mind's eye, you might be able to picture this buffet lunch or a similar situation in which you could be prone to overeat certain foods, particularly high-sugar or ultra-processed foods. These foods are so uniquely alluring because they trigger a 'hit' or 'high' through the rush of a brain chemical (neurotransmitter) called dopamine. The part of your brain where these dopamine pleasure messages are transmitted is known as your reward centre. This is the same part of your brain that is stimulated by drugs like cocaine and amphetamine.

Dopamine generates feelings of pleasure in your brain by attaching to a receptor called the dopamine-D2-receptor. Your genes control the number of dopamine receptors in your reward centre and you might have genes that programme you to have fewer dopamine-D2-receptors than other people. The upshot of this is that when you eat high-sugar foods, dopamine cannot generate as much of a pleasure rush in your brain because it has fewer receptors to attach to. This blunted dopamine pleasure hit might lead you to overeat sugary, ultra-processed foods to compensate for the dulled dopamine effect.

You might recognize yourself in this scenario, where you eat sweet foods and you get a pleasure high but it's not quite enough – you are experiencing a few fireworks when what you're looking for is a full technicolour display. So you go back for more, seeking out that elusive hit, which the reduced numbers of dopamine-D2-receptors in your brain's reward centre are failing to ignite.

By understanding how your genes influence your response to these sorts of foods, I hope you can let go of the idea that, with enough willpower, you will be able to eat just a small amount. Instead, as my patients have done, you can choose to use this self-knowledge to make food choices that keep you in control of your eating.

How do I know if my weight gain is down to my genes?

Variations in dopamine pleasure signalling and the FTO gene are two examples of how your own unique set of genes can contribute to the tendency to be a certain weight. Scientists call this your 'gene burden score' – the risk written into your genes for gaining weight.

Some of my patients have wondered about their own genetic predisposition to weight gain and exactly which versions of these weight-influencing genes they have. It is possible to enrol in a research study or even to pay a commercial company to sequence your genes to generate your personal gene burden score. However, such an approach is rarely necessary because the answer can often be found in your eating history. Research shows that a high gene burden score for weight gain tends to first declare itself in childhood, manifesting in a blunted or dulled feeling of fullness, which can lead to overeating. So if you tended to want seconds of birthday cake at childhood tea parties and your favourite part of breakfast was scraping the last crystals of sugar from the bottom of the cereal bowl, then you may well have a high gene burden score. The scientific analysis would likely simply confirm what your memories have already told you.

You and your thrifty genes

Before you put in a call to your parents to lodge a complaint about the genes that they have passed on to you, it is worthwhile bearing in mind that there are clear biological reasons why so many of us have been dealt a genetic hand that gives us some degree of risk when it comes to weight gain. These pro-weight-gain genes made us the survivors.

Throughout most of history, the key challenge for humans has been a lack of food, not an overabundance of it. This is why, over tens of thousands of years, we have evolved genes that promote weight gain. For millennia, carrying these genes gave our ancestors an advantage because when they did spear a buffalo or find fruit on the trees, they gained weight easily and had plentiful fat stores for a rainy day. As a result, they were more likely to survive the famine than someone who remained lean. This weight-gain advantage meant that they went on to reproduce, passing the genes associated with weight gain on to the next generation.

From an evolutionary standpoint, it would also have been advantageous to have genes that make our brains particularly drawn to sugary foods. The desire for a sweet hit would have spurred on our ancestors to search out the last fruits on the blackberry bush despite the brambles and to climb the tree to steal the bees' honey regardless of the stings.

It's only with the development of the modern food landscape that these weight-gain genes, which served us well for thousands of years, have become a distinct disadvantage.

The clue is in your family photo album

When I was a child, one of my favourite pastimes was looking through our family photo albums. Precious photographs from the 1970s, with their neat square shape and rounded corners, capturing birthdays, day trips to the seaside, new babies and sometimes no occasion at all. Then, it was the clothes and the hairstyles and the cars that fascinated me. Now, as I turn the pages, one other thing strikes me. Almost nobody in these photographs had a weight issue.

If you have a family album from this era, you will certainly also make the same observation. Yet the people in these photographs had the same pro-weight-gain genes as us (as did their parents, grandparents and so on).

To put this into context, in the 1970s, about 7 per cent of the country were, by medical definition, classified as obese. This figure has quadrupled in a generation – today obesity affects more than one in four adults with a further 36 per cent classified as overweight. Taken together, two-thirds of us now have a weight problem. Yet almost everyone in those 1970s photographs was lean.

Something has profoundly changed. And it isn't our genes.

A journey back in time to a world that kept us lean

The photographs were taken in a food landscape that has become almost unrecognizable to us today, and one in which our weight-control genes didn't work against us. In the 1970s, one of the barriers to overeating was the cost of food. Back then, food was expensive, accounting for 25 per cent of household spending, costing more than housing and utilities combined. This meant that, for most people, food could not be over-purchased, so the amount bought usually matched our body's requirements.

Things are very different today. Food is generally cheaper and more widely available, so we spend just 10 per cent of our earnings on food. As a result, many more people now live with food security. We should of course celebrate this, but there is a caveat – many of today's foods, particularly ultra-processed foods, can provide us with fuel, but these same foods are usually high in sugar, low in fibre and are of poor quality. So while we now have food security, we do not have nutritional security.

In the 1970s, retail practices also limited food availability. Grocers and supermarkets had shorter opening hours. Many shops still had half-day closing midweek and by law, there was no Sunday trading. So meals had to be planned ahead and food bought during time-limited opening hours. This was normal. If we didn't buy food when the shops were open, the fridge was empty and we couldn't solve this by eating out, because going to a restaurant was an expensive, infrequent treat. Fast food was only just starting to arrive on the high street and doorstep delivery was still at least a decade away.

By necessity (if not also by choice), we had to cook, rarely eating food prepared outside the home. Ultra-processed food was beginning to find its way into our kitchens in the form of freeze-dried mashed potatoes and powdered, just-add-milk desserts. However, these foods made up far less than the 50 per cent of our diet that they do today (more on this in the next chapter). Instead, we usually cooked from scratch and we understood the majority of the ingredients we were using within a trusted (and often more limited) repertoire of meals.

In the world of the now-faded photographs, there were also social norms and expectations about when to eat and when not to eat. On the whole, eating took place at a table, usually with other people. This was the world of an older generation who frowned upon eating on public transport or while walking along the street. Eating usually happened at set, defined mealtimes. We then waited until the next meal to eat again, affording us Eating Window micro-closures (see page 61), although, of course, we didn't call it this – all we were doing was not eating between meals. Snacking had yet to become a familiar word, pushed by the food industry to convince us to eat frequently to sustain us through the day, while at the same time profiting from our permanently open Eating Window.

Back in the days of the photographs, our biology had not been hijacked by constant sugar consumption. Not only was blood sugar running stable (the blood-sugar rollercoaster had not yet come to town), but the brain's reward centre was not being relentlessly assaulted by a sugar-induced dopamine hit. Sugar was part of the diet, but it was not the mainstay. A slice of birthday cake or an ice cream on holiday were treats, not everyday items. Some of the people in the photographs might have had weight-gain genes like FTO Risk, but because sugary, ultra-processed foods were not eaten every day, trying to limit their consumption was not a constant struggle.

If we could have frozen time in the 1970s, I think weight issues would have remained unusual. The people from the photo album had the same weight-gain genes as we do, but they nevertheless remained lean. Their slim appearance was not down to home chefs, personal trainers, specialist knowledge or unusual resources. Rather, they were regular everyday people who simply lived in a food landscape that suited their genes.

The good news here is that these photographs show us that our genes do not doom us to a certain weight destiny. Instead, we can think of our weight-gain genes as the loaded gun. It is the modern harmful food environment that pulls the trigger. We cannot change our genes, but we can work with them. The loaded gun is simply a risk. If you choose to use Programme tools like food choices and an Eating Window, you will be eating in a way that your genes are suited to. By living in this way, just as we did in the past, the loaded weight-gain gene gun remains of no consequence, because you are choosing not to pull the trigger.

CHOICES

Choice 1: Choose not to pull the trigger

As we've seen, your genes are not your fate. They simply mean that you are better suited to some environments than others.

Let's look at the example of skin colour to illustrate this. Your genes determine your skin colour. If you have pale-skin genes, you are unsuited to being in intensely sunny places. You can decide to ignore this or hope to override your genes and go out in the midday sun, but then you risk getting sunburnt and even potentially developing skin cancer. Instead, most people with pale-skin genes choose to protect themselves from an environment (bright sunshine) that their genes make them unsuited to – they might wear a hat, use high-factor sunblock, seek out shade and avoid going out at the sunniest time of day.

It isn't possible, as one private individual, for you to change today's harmful food environment. But you can choose to protect yourself from it. Just as someone who has pale-skin genes will protect themselves against the sun, if you have weight-gain genes, you can protect yourself by turning back the clock to live in the world of the photographs.

You can do this by using your Programme tools, such as

choosing to know your ingredients and cooking and eating food that your body recognizes as food. You can also choose to avoid sugar and foods that the body very quickly breaks down into sugar. And you can choose to have an Eating Window. By using all of these tools together, you are stepping into a time machine that takes you back to a world that suits your genes, empowering you to take control of your weight whatever genes you may have inherited.

This is what my patient Mital – whose enriching words open this chapter – chose to do. Mital asked herself questions about the likely genetic hand that she had been dealt. She recognized how certain foods manipulated her brain's reward centre – 'I used to be so jealous of people who could say no to chocolate or open a pack of biscuits and not finish it all.' This self-knowledge was empowering for Mital and she decided there were certain foods that she would never be able to control, so it was better to avoid them altogether. Rather than fight her biology, Mital chose to protect herself from these foods – 'Now I don't even want that stuff in my home!'

You can do this too. When you ask questions and make decisions about the weight-control genes that you might have, you too will live in the food landscape of the photographs, where the characters, looking out in their cravats, bell-bottoms and platform shoes, were in control of their eating and stayed lean, even though they had the same weight-gain genes as us.

Choice 2: Reintroducing certain foods –
how do I tailor the Programme to my genes?

The chapters in this book mirror my patients' fortnightly group sessions, and so by the time we get to Session 7, fourteen weeks into the Programme, my patients start to ask, 'When could I choose to reintroduce . . . ?' (see pages 23–4 and 201–2). What they mean by this is, 'I'm following the Programme and things are ticking along nicely. At some point in the future, I might like to have a piece of toast with my eggs or a pudding at a celebratory meal.'

This is how I answer this question.

We don't know the exact genetic hand you have been dealt, so it will be a trial and error approach, as everyone's response to these foods will be unique. For example, if you and your partner are following the Programme together, your responses to reintroducing certain foods will be different because you have different genes.

Perhaps in the future, your partner will find that they can eat dessert after a special meal and this doesn't trigger overeating or stall their weight loss. On the other hand, you might eat the dessert and it sets off some dopamine fireworks but not quite the hit you were looking for, driving you towards eating another helping and then another in a search for the full pleasure high. At the end of the experiment, you might conclude that eating dessert occasionally is suitable for your partner, but that it simply doesn't work with the wiring of your brain's reward centre. Just as Mital did, this self-awareness might lead you to conclude that there are certain foods that you can't control and you may want to completely exclude them for the long term.

But we're also talking about the good news in this chapter, which means you might find that reintroducing other foods works well for you. You could add some roast potatoes now and again with your Sunday lunch or perhaps occasionally have a slice of toast with your eggs. These will taste good to you, but you will be able to eat them in a controlled way and move on without impacting on your weight.

What's fascinating is that many of my patients enjoy the 'When could I choose to reintroduce . . . ?' discussion that we have at Session 7, and they hold that knowledge close, yet even many years down the line, they still choose not to change very much. For the first time, they have found a way of eating that works for them. They feel good, they have reversed their health issues and are at a weight that they want to be. Rather than missing the old foods, in fact, like Mital, they identify that although they had eaten these foods for years leading up to the Programme, these foods weren't working with their unique set of genes.

Through the Programme, my patients find foods that suit their biology, and this feels good. They have re-engaged with a way of eating that has suited humans for generations, and that suits them too. This means the loaded genetic gun is of no consequence because through their food choices – although the gun is loaded – the safety catch stays on.

Like my patients, I hope that you too can use this self-knowledge to protect yourself from the ultra-processed foods that dominate today's food landscape. With your new understanding that our biology isn't suited to this way of eating, it's time for the next chapter – the food industry.

CHAPTER 8

The food industry

'I am no longer living a sugar-fuelled life
and it feels amazing! I honestly felt like
I had not been conscious for years, and
not only is this improving my physical
health but mentally I am now so much
more in control than I have ever been.'
Alice, lost 3 stone 11lb (24kg)

The next time you go to a supermarket, if you pause and take a look around, you'll notice that a vast proportion of the food on offer is ultra-processed. Rows of shelves stacked high with industrially produced bread, colourful sweetened yogurts, reconstituted meat products, ready meals, breakfast cereal, stir-in sauces, soft drinks, confectionery, biscuits and puddings. The seeming abundance of thousands of different products gives us the illusion of choice when in reality these foods are simply various combinations of the same few ingredients: sugar, salt, poor-quality fats, artificial sweeteners, emulsifiers, preservatives and other additives.

This chapter will explain how, if you have struggled to

make healthy food choices in the past, this is not your fault. Like the rest of us, you have been caught up in the grasp of the food industry – large, smart, rich corporations that are called 'Big Food' by some scientists.

You can think of today's food landscape as being like a sickly fairground merry-go-round ride. When we first get on to the ride, we are buying ultra-processed food because Big Food makes this way of eating seem like the default or even the 'normal' option. As the ride goes round, we might feel giddy, nauseous or unwell and want to get off. But this food has been meticulously engineered by food scientists to ensure that we can't stop eating it. We are now trapped on the ultra-processed food merry-go-round, unable to control our consumption because this food has hacked our brain's biology, making us need more and more of it.

As always with the Programme, this chapter is not simply about calling out problems. Rather, it will give you the science that explains the serious impact that ultra-processed food has on your weight and health and will support you with strategies for getting off this sickly food merry-go-round. By turning your back on Big Food and its tricks, you can instead choose to embrace the wealth of flavours, joy and health benefits of eating real food.

What is processed and ultra-processed food?

The first step towards rejecting ultra-processed food is to understand what these foods are. The terms 'processed' and 'ultra-processed' – as well as other descriptions you might have heard of, like 'unprocessed' or 'minimally processed' – were devised by scientists to describe the nature and extent of processing that the food has undergone.

Unprocessed or minimally processed foods include eggs, milk, natural yogurt, meat, fish and seafood, nuts and seeds, fruit and vegetables, and herbs and spices. These are one ingredient foods, which have been eaten by humans for thousands of years.

Processed foods are made by adding sugar, oil, salt and other substances to food to increase shelf-life and to enhance the sensory experience of eating the food. Examples include fruit in syrup, sugared nuts and tinned vegetables preserved in sugar and salt water.

Ultra-processed foods (UPF) are foods that have undergone intensive industrial processing (hence ultra-processed) that has no equivalent techniques in home cooking. Examples of ultra-processing include hydrogenation and other chemical processes like extrusion, moulding and pre-frying. UPF uses low-cost, high-margin ingredients not found in a domestic kitchen, such as anti-foaming agents, high-fructose corn syrup and soya protein isolate. Artificial sweeteners, flavourings, dyes, thickeners, bulking agents and emulsifiers are added to give the food a deeply alluring quality, while also disguising unpleasant colours, smells or textures arising from the ingredients and the processing.

For the rest of this chapter, we'll be particularly looking at UPF because these are the foods that are most devastating to health and weight control.

What's wrong with ultra-processed food?

It can be easy to think of UPF – foods like biscuits, fizzy drinks, sweets and crisps – as being bad for us simply because they contain 'empty calories', but this idea has now been over-taken by a recent game-changing experiment. Under careful observation, research participants ate only UPF for two weeks – foods like white-bread sandwiches, diet fizzy drinks and ready meals – followed by two weeks of eating only un-processed foods like baked cod, almonds and blueberries. Importantly, the two diets contained the same number of cal-ories, and subjects were allowed to eat as much or as little of the allocated food as they liked. Both diets were also matched for sugar, fat, salt and fibre content (although the fibre in the UPF diet had to be given as a supplement because UPF is so inherently low in fibre). Researchers found that when eating the UPF diet, the participants overate by 500 calories a day and gained almost a kilogram (2 pounds) in two weeks. When they switched to the unprocessed diet, they naturally ate less and lost the weight they had gained.

So if it's not the calories in UPF, then why are these foods so bad for us? Breaking UPF down into its component parts shows us that these foods have a number of common features. Lack of fibre starves the gut-bacteria workforce and a low protein content fails to generate the fullness hormone text messages that we need to prevent weight gain. Large amounts of salt guarantee a long shelf-life, and cheap, poor-quality, synthetic fats, including trans fats, add to palatability but are associated with cardiovascular diseases such as heart attacks.

Additives are routinely included, such as food colourings like Sunset Yellow (E110), which has been linked to hyperactivity in children (foods containing E110 now come with a safety warning on the label for this additive). Lastly, there's the trump card in the food industry's hand, the one that is found in almost all UPF: sugar. Sugar tips us into fat-storage mode (high levels of insulin – broom out, sweeping) and traps us on the blood-sugar rollercoaster. And it's the sugar that keeps us hooked.

The great biology hack

If you find it difficult to stop eating UPF like biscuits, crisps, fizzy drinks and ice cream, this has nothing to do with a lack of willpower and everything to do with how these foods have been engineered to hack your biology.

The food industry spends millions on scientists and food engineers who carefully design every part of the eating experience, then repeatedly test their products in food-tasting focus groups. The food must have a very particular texture and consistency ('mouth-feel') and is usually formulated to dissolve in the mouth. These foods are designed to be easy to eat, slipping down with a minimal requirement for chewing. In fact, if you hold UPF in your mouth for long enough, it is usually possible, like baby food, to eventually swallow it without any chewing at all – sliced white bread, biscuits, breakfast cereal and crisps being some common examples.

Most importantly, these foods are designed to act on the brain's reward centre. As we discussed in the last chapter, the reward centre is the part of the brain where we experience pleasure through a rush of the brain chemical dopamine. The reward centre is the same part of the brain that is stimulated when people take a drug like cocaine.

In fact, research suggests that sweet taste might be even more alluring than cocaine, with laboratory rats choosing to drink sweetened water over a hit of intravenous cocaine when given a choice between the two. It's no wonder that once you start eating sugary UPF like ice cream or biscuits, it's hard to stop.

The food industry's skill in generating a powerful dopamine high explains the paradox of why we continue to buy and eat UPF despite knowing the negative consequences. This is backed up by scientific research. In one important study, laboratory rats trained to expect an electric shock in association with eating UPF like cake and chocolate nevertheless kept on eating it despite the threat of the shock. You might think that this is scientifically interesting, but we humans don't get electric shocks if we eat UPF. Except we do. In contrast to the experimental rats, our electric shocks are weight gain, diabetes, heart disease, acid reflux, energy slumps and the numerous other consequences of eating these foods. And just like the rats, we are prepared to pay a high price for continued consumption and for the fleeting high of the dopamine pleasure rush.

Is ultra-processed food addictive?

There is an ongoing medical and academic debate about whether UPF, and sugar in particular, is addictive. The American Psychiatric Association's criteria for the diagnosis of addiction include cravings or the intense urge to use the substance, continued use despite harmful consequences and repeated attempts to quit. Whether, as a technical matter, UPF and sugar are ultimately found to meet the criteria for addiction, this story of use and despair is one that many of my patients would have recognized before joining the Programme.

Inconvenience food

It's not just the food scientists and engineers that have pushed UPF into our kitchens. They have been amply supported by Big Food's powerfully persuasive marketing messages that have told us a story – that we are busy and we have no time. We have no time to plan and shop and chop and stir. So to help us out, the food industry promises us 'convenience' – selling us foods that will make our lives easier.

The advertising message is that these foods relieve us from having to plan ahead, buy ingredients and 'waste' time cooking. What's more, this industrially produced, usually long-life food will be ready quickly. Perhaps it takes just four minutes in the microwave or a few seconds to add boiling water or maybe no preparation is needed at all. We are encouraged not to carry our own home-prepared food because of the readily available UPF that we can grab and go from any supermarket, coffee shop or petrol station.

We know, however, that UPF is in fact 'inconvenience' food: eating it results in weight gain and type 2 diabetes, as well as the daily discomfort of bloating, headaches, lack of energy and low mood. It's inconvenient to worry about what to wear and where to shop for clothes. It's inconvenient to be nervous about social occasions. It's inconvenient to feel low and lacking in confidence. It's inconvenient to be uneasy around certain people who might make unkind comments. And it's inconvenient to use your precious time on doctors' appointments and pharmacy visits.

The idea of 'convenience' food has tricked us out of cooking for ourselves from scratch, using ingredients that we understand and that have been eaten by human beings for centuries. Cooking is such a fundamental life skill that it is included in the Activities of Daily Living, a list of medically defined self-care tasks that you must be capable of in order to lead an independent life. The Activities of Daily Living include showering, going to the bathroom, mobility, managing your own money – and cooking. If we don't cook for ourselves, we become dependent on the food industry to feed us, eroding our independence and reducing our quality of life.

But we have choices. It's time to take back control.

CHOICES

Choice 1: Be vigilant for UPF
ingredients that pretend to be food

The first step in turning your back on UPF is to know how to recognize it. Unlike cigarette packets, these foods are not mandated to come with warnings on the label or photographs of their devastating health consequences. Instead, you will need to check the ingredients carefully and if you see any of the following, it's a red-flag that this food is UPF:

> Acidity Regulator, Anti-foaming Agents, Artificial Sweeteners (these often include sweeteners such as Sucralose, Aspartame and Acesulfame-K), Colours, Emulsifiers (Soya Lecithin and mono- and diglycerides of fatty acids are common), Firming Agents, Humectants, Hydrogenated Oils, Hydrolyzed Protein, Maltodextrin, Modified Starches, Preservatives, Soy Protein Isolate, Sugar and sugar by another name (for example, Dextrose, Fruit Juice Concentrate, High-fructose Corn Syrup – also called Glucose-fructose Syrup and Invert Sugar), Whey Protein

This is not an exhaustive list, so if you come across a dubious-sounding ingredient that is not mentioned here, ask yourself these three questions to check if it is a health-sapping UPF:

1. **Can I pronounce this ingredient?**
   For example, in our groups we find mono- and diacetyl tartaric acid esters of mono- and diglycerides of fatty acids particularly tricky.

2. **Do I understand what this ingredient is?**
   Using the above example, with a PhD from Imperial College and in all the years of running the Programme, I still couldn't tell you with any degree of confidence or precision what mono- and diacetyl tartaric acid esters of mono- and diglycerides of fatty acids actually are.

3. **Is this an ingredient that a home cook would have in their kitchen?**
   I have yet to hear a Programme participant tell me that they keep stearoyl-2-lactylate or sulphur dioxide in their store cupboard.

Finally, picturing the following scenario is a good litmus test for deciding whether an ingredient is likely to be healthy or harmful. Imagine you are caring for a baby. That baby trusts you to nurture her and to make choices about her food that will keep her healthy and strong. Can you imagine spooning acesulfame-K or soya lecithin into her mouth? I know even the thought of it would make you shudder. So in the same way that we nurture and look after those we love, it is time to afford yourself that same care. These ingredients are not the right fuel for your body. They are synthetic, industrially produced chemicals masquerading as food, which cause weight gain and health problems and which do not support your body to run in top condition. Be kind to yourself. You deserve better.

Choice 2: Choose not to eat foods with (many) ingredients

Choice 1 allows you to quickly spot if a food is UPF. But if you look back to the Choose to Eat List on pages 20–2, you'll see that our Programme food choices fit neatly into the best and healthiest category – unprocessed or minimally processed foods. These are wholefoods that don't come with a list of ingredients. When you buy broccoli, there are no ingredients. It's broccoli. The same applies to, for example, eggs, chicken, milk and strawberries. These are the foods that humans were designed to eat – no ingredients, no tricks.

If you do buy a pre-prepared food that has some ingredients, like mayonnaise or hummus, it will be better if there are very few ingredients and that they are recognizable, natural foods. For example, hummus should contain chickpeas, tahini, olive oil, lemon juice, garlic and salt.

Choice 3: Be prepared

We live in an environment where the 'normal' is to eat poor-quality, high-sugar, industrially produced UPF. This means that when you are away from home, at work or out for the day, it is hard, without some forward planning, to eat well.

Even if you live in a big city, it's rare that good-quality, nutritious, healthy food is easily available. Choose not to entrust your health and wellbeing to big multinational corporations, fast-food chains and coffee shops. If you do this, you are playing a game of roulette with your weight and health and remember, the house always wins . . .

Instead, be prepared and carry your own packed food with you. My patients report that the delicious Programme packed lunch they take to work attracts envious looks while their colleagues tuck into mass-produced sandwiches and crisps. What's more, carrying your own food will save you money – often in excess of £10 a day compared to buying lunch and snacks from coffee shops and other outlets.

Choice 4: Take back control of your plate – choose to eat the real convenience foods

You can choose to close the book on the 'no time to cook' story by deciding that the food industry will not manipulate you into giving up cooking. You can take a stand against the message that their sugar-filled, synthetic products are superior to the food that you can prepare from scratch and that your body recognizes as food. Your home-cooked food is delicious, nourishing and does not hack your biology. Instead, it feeds your gut bacteria, triggers fullness hormone text messages and is coloured by health-giving phytonutrients rather than artificial chemicals. The food you cook tastes good but does not exploit your reward centre and you can easily choose to stop eating it if you want to.

This is what my patient Alice – whose inspiring words open the chapter – chose to do. After years of eating an ultra-processed diet – 'I honestly felt like I had not been conscious for years' – Alice joined the Programme and chose to shut out the food industry. She concluded that it was impossible to control eating foods that are deliberately engineered to target her brain's reward centre. Instead, Alice chose to cook and enjoy all the delicious Programme 'convenience' foods that allowed her to reclaim her health – 'I am no longer living a sugar-fuelled life and it feels amazing! . . . Not only is this improving my physical health but mentally I am now so much more in control than I have ever been.'

What Alice understood is that willpower and self-discipline will never be enough to overcome the pleasure effect that UPF has on the brain, but instead, that liberation from overeating comes from choosing to reject these ultra-processed foods.

Choice 5: Choose to create your own new normal

UPF is so embedded in the modern food landscape that eating it is considered to be 'normal'. Except, of course, there is a very knowledgeable group of people – my patients and you, the readers of this book – who do not find this normal at all. What an amazing position for you to be in. Sometimes it can feel uncomfortable or challenging to make food choices that fall outside what is considered 'normal'. But once you dare to be different, you will find – as my patients do – that fortune favours the brave.

Just as the perception of smoking has gone from fashionable and desirable to unpleasant and stigmatized within a generation, the tide is turning on UPF and you are at the vanguard of this. In 1950, scientists first showed that cigarette smoking causes lung cancer. Yet it still took a further fifty-seven years after the original research study before smoking was banned in all public indoor spaces – in 2007.

The progress that we have made on smoking is a cause for hope. But as the smoking story shows us, social norms and government regulation take time to catch up with the science.

The science on UPF's devastating health effects is here now. You don't need to wait for wider societal attitudes to catch up with this knowledge or for UPF to become more tightly regulated by new laws. By following the Programme and rejecting UPF and Big Food, you are taking your own action. You are protecting yourself from tricks and hacks and you are reclaiming your health and wellbeing. At some point, eating UPF will no longer be considered normal. Until then, we can make our own choices to take back control and we can create our own new normal.

CHAPTER 9

History lessons

'What the Programme has done is empower me
to make choices about my life and health. It has
given me a language and tools to challenge myself.
I have the ownership. There is still work for me
to do, and I will always have to be careful not to
fall back into old habits, but I can now choose to
treat myself rather than get sicker and rely on the
NHS to deal with the results. For the first time I
understand why I got sick, why I ate the way I did
and that I could choose to do something about it.'
Richard, lost 3 stone 9lb (23kg)

There are certain health conditions like weight gain, diabetes and high blood pressure that are now so common it
can be easy for us to accept them as inevitable, even 'normal'.
But we only need to take a small step back in time to see
that these problems are not an expected or unavoidable part
of the human condition. Instead, there was a time, in living
memory, when weight issues and associated illnesses like diabetes were unusual, even rare.

This chapter is about suggesting a mindset shift that reframes these conditions from health problems that many people have become resigned to having, to an awareness that they are in fact a consequence of the lifestyle choices that we make. Like my patients, I hope that you will find this a hopeful, good news message because your lifestyle choices are of course directly within your control. Rather than accepting weight gain and associated health problems as inevitable, this chapter will show you that instead you have the agency to choose a life that is full of good health, living at a weight that is right for you.

Many of these lifestyle choices will be similar to those that were common in the recent past, at a time when it was normal to maintain a healthy weight, free of health problems like diabetes. By learning the lessons of history, it is possible for us to live this way too.

Life on the home front – the health of the nation

At the stroke of midnight on 5 July 1948, an institution was born that would become the most loved and trusted in our national life. Famously described as 'the closest thing the English have to a religion', the National Health Service (NHS) was established to provide universal 'cradle to grave' medical care, free at the point of delivery, with access determined by clinical need and not the ability to pay.

Founded just after the end of World War Two, the NHS was established at a time when weight problems and conditions like type 2 diabetes, which had not been common, had become rarer still as a consequence of government policy during the war.

During World War Two, most foods were rationed – except fruit, vegetables, fish and bread (although white bread was prohibited). Contrary to what you might expect, rationing saw significant improvements in both nutritional quality and quantity for many people. The Dig for Victory scheme encouraged people to grow their own vegetables; and the Ministry of Information urged people not to overserve themselves, with the public health message: 'Don't take more than you can eat.'

Petrol rationing was introduced within weeks of the outbreak of war and then, in 1942, it was withdrawn from the public altogether, reserved for official use only. Civilian car use (for those who had them) stopped entirely, which meant that all journeys had to be made by bicycle, public transport or preferably on foot. 'Walk short distances,' the public was told, 'and leave room for those who have longer journeys.'

Although these measures were introduced as part of the war effort on the home front, food rationing, care with portion sizes and increased amounts of physical exercise were to have a significant and unforeseen outcome: cases of type 2 diabetes fell sharply and, in the years immediately following the war, diabetes appeared to be a disease in decline. Set against a backdrop of the conquering of infectious diseases by antibiotics and childhood vaccinations, a new 'Golden Age' of medicine was emerging. And at the centre of this Golden Age shone our new Health Service, with a mission that emphasized 'the promotion of good health rather than only the treatment of bad'. This was to be a National Health Service, not a National Disease Service. With the end of the war and advances in medicine and surgery promising a brighter tomorrow, there was a surge of optimism that things (and people's health) could only get better.

What happened to the Golden Age?

Nobody at the time, not the doctors nor the scientists nor the politicians, saw the storm of weight gain and diabetes that was coming just over the horizon. Nobody could have predicted that our diets would become far less healthy than during the years of rationing. Nobody foresaw the 140 teaspoons of sugar a week that would become the normal way of eating. Nobody predicted that the food industry would trick its way into our kitchens and on to our plates. Nobody anticipated that, with the return of fuel to civilian use, driving would become the default mode of travel, even for short journeys. Nobody could have known that people would spend all day being still, with life coming to them through a screen. Nobody could have expected sleep deprivation to become such a common part of everyday life.

By the early 1990s, far from the promise and optimism of the Golden Age, the NHS found itself looking after a population that was, in fact, getting sicker. While in the founding years of the NHS, type 2 diabetes had been beaten into retreat by food rationing and more physical activity, this disease has now come to dominate the modern Health Service.

Today, one in fifteen of us in the UK (4.7 million people)

has diabetes. That's a number that has more than doubled over the last twenty years. Nine in ten cases are type 2 diabetes, which is closely associated with excess weight. The textbooks I read at medical school describe type 2 diabetes as a disease of older people – this has since been updated. Type 2 diabetes is being diagnosed younger and younger and is now even affecting children.

The NHS increasingly struggles to shoulder the case numbers and the associated costs. Every year the NHS spends £10 billion, or 10 per cent of its entire budget, on diabetes alone. This equates to diabetes costing the NHS £19,000 a minute or over £1,000,000 an hour. Experts now worry about the potential for diabetes to 'bankrupt' the NHS. An institution so loved that in the spring of 2020, at the height of the Covid-19 pandemic, we stood on our doorsteps and clapped for it, is at risk of sinking under the rising tide of an illness that in the 1940s seemed to be all but disappearing.

Something has gone terribly wrong.

'It's just one of those things . . . '

By looking back just eighty years, we can see that neither weight gain, diabetes nor any other associated health conditions are inevitable. We know this because in the recent past, when we ate and moved in a different way, hardly anyone had these conditions that are now considered to be 'normal'.

My patients tell me that by understanding this historical context, they can see that their weight or health problems are not inevitable, but in fact can be traced back to major societal shifts – from the devastation of the food landscape by ultra-processed food to modern life allowing for hours of stillness.

Although they weren't expecting a history lesson when they joined the Programme, they discover that by looking to the past, they find answers to the question that so many had asked for years about their weight and health: 'Why . . . ?'

'Why does my weight continue to go up?' 'Why do I have diabetes or high blood pressure or sleep apnoea or fatty liver or acid reflux?' 'Why am I bloated or uncomfortable after eating?' 'Why am I always tired?'

Until they started on the Programme, many of my patients had been unable to find a satisfactory answer to these questions, so instead they concluded that, 'It's just one of those things.'

In our groups, when this comes up we look at things in a different way. Rather than having a weight or health issue, we discuss the scenario of having a maintenance problem at home, say a broken boiler or a leaking roof. Imagine that someone comes to take a look and then presents you with a large bill. When you ask, 'Why has this problem occurred?' you are told, 'It's just one of those things . . .'

I suspect that you wouldn't find this explanation at all satisfactory, yet many of us have resigned ourselves to the idea that problems with our weight and health are 'just one of those things'. It's not only the science that you have learnt in this book that gives you the confidence to know that this conclusion is incorrect. We also know this because, as recently as eighty years ago, hardly anyone had weight issues and associated health conditions that are now considered to be 'just one of those things'.

A step back in time to the Blue Zones

There are certain places around the world where, in comparison to our 'modern' lives, time has stood still. People who live in these so-called 'Blue Zones' – Ikaria, Greece; Loma Linda, USA; Nicoya, Costa Rica; Sardinia, Italy; and Okinawa, Japan – have some of the longest life expectancies in the world. Blue Zones do not have state-of-the-art hospitals or treatments and medications that the rest of us don't have access to. Instead, it is their lack of 'progress' – eating traditional, unprocessed diets and being physically active – that makes them so remarkable. And it is by holding on to their historical lifestyle and traditions that Blue Zone populations live long, healthy lives, with unusually low levels of diabetes or weight gain.

Addressing the root cause – not papering over the cracks

When we re-frame illnesses like weight gain, diabetes or high blood pressure as being a consequence of our lifestyle choices, then it gives us the agency to make decisions to address the root cause of these health issues. For some of my patients, this is a new and exciting way of thinking, because prior to this they had believed the only solution was to take medication. The issue here is that while medications can manage the symptoms, they cannot address the root cause of why these illnesses developed in the first place.

To help understand the difference between tackling the root cause of a condition and treating the symptoms, let's look at the example of smoking. Imagine you are a cigarette smoker and your health is suffering – let's say you are breathless and you have a cough. If we take the approach of treating the symptoms, then at a hypothetical doctor's visit you would be given an inhaler to help with the breathing difficulties while you carried on smoking. If instead we address the root cause, the doctor would, in addition to treating your symptoms, offer to help you quit smoking.

The first approach, using an inhaler and continuing to smoke, is like applying wallpaper over the cracks in a wall without treating the subsidence that's causing those cracks in the first place.

It's exactly the same with eating an ultra-processed, high-sugar, low-fibre diet. Just like smoking, these foods take your health. The solution to the damage caused by these foods is the same as our smoking example. When you look upstream of the symptoms (weight gain, diabetes) to the root cause of the problem (these harmful foods), we can see that the best treatment is to quit those foods – just like giving up smoking. Not searching for a 'pill for every ill'; not papering over the cracks.

'I have the ownership'

Tackling the cause of his health problems head-on is exactly what my patient Richard did, whose thoughtful reflections open this chapter. Richard had been diagnosed with type 2 diabetes two years before starting the Programme. Having been told that diabetes was a lifelong condition, Richard had resigned himself to this. When he started the Programme he was presented with all of the choices that you have read about and he decided to chart his own future – 'I have the ownership.'

Richard joined the Programme, lost 3 stone 9lb (23kg) and four years later remains free from diabetes and off medication. Richard felt that the right to free and universal healthcare comes with responsibilities. Empowered by his Programme knowledge, as Richard says, he made the choice, 'to treat myself rather than get sicker and rely on the NHS to deal with the results'.

Richard is rightly proud that his choices have freed up precious time and money that will 'protect the NHS', just as we were asked to do during the Covid-19 pandemic. With more Richards supported to make similar decisions, the future of the NHS could be increasingly protected with the potential to be a Health Service, true to the vision of its original architects.

Like Richard, you too now understand the science and the history and so his words can become yours too – 'For the first time I understand why I got sick, why I ate the way I did and that I could choose to do something about it.'

Using your Programme tools to address the root cause of your weight gain and health issues

The aim of this chapter is not to give you any new choices. Instead, it is intended to show you that there was a time, in the not too distant past, when people ate and moved in a way that is similar to the Programme choices you have already read about. This way of living allowed them to lead healthy lives free from weight gain, and this way of living is one that you can adopt yourself in our modern age.

If you have health conditions, please never stop medications or change your treatment plan without speaking to your doctor. Instead, like my own patients have done, you can work with your doctor using your Programme choices, towards a shared goal of stopping particular tablets and improving, or even reversing, certain health conditions.

Before we move on to the next chapters, which explore themes around mindset and behaviour change, here is a reminder of all the powerful Programme tools in your toolkit so far:

1. Choosing to eat food that is delicious and nutritious while at the same time lowering insulin levels, transforming you into an efficient fat-burning machine.
2. Listening to your body's brilliant hunger–fullness signalling system so that you eat when you are hungry and you stop when you are full. ('I don't have hunger.')

3. Choosing the opening and closing times of your Eating Window, perhaps opting for eight hours open and sixteen hours closed.

4. Nourishing your gut bacteria so that it works to keep you lean.

5. Choosing to keep moving every single day, committing to never short-changing yourself by being still.

6. Prioritizing sleep as the ultimate restorative reset and avoiding the hormonal storm of sleep deprivation, which will drive weight gain.

7. Understanding that your weight-gain genes are the loaded gun and that, by protecting yourself from the modern, harmful food environment, you are choosing not to pull the trigger.

8. Choosing to avoid ultra-processed food that's full of sugar and dubious ingredients, which hack your biology and are very difficult to control.

Science can sometimes seem slightly abstract, so I hope that looking at things through this historical prism gives you a real-life context to all the new science you are reading about. Against this background, this chapter frames how you can use your tools as a powerful way to address the root cause of weight gain and its associated health issues. Now that you know these conditions are not 'just one of those things', your Programme tools will put you in the driving seat. You have the 'ownership'.

CHAPTER 10

Language

'I'm thinking about that very first session and the long road to knowledge and recovery we embarked on that day. We have come a long and rich way from despair to enlightenment, from the impossible to the possible. Thank you for it all.'

Meriem, lost 3 stone 7lb (22kg)

The words that you use when you speak to yourself are the most powerful words you hear because they will shape your beliefs and your beliefs shape your outcomes. You might think, that can't be right, what my boss or my partner or my friends say to me is far more influential than the conversations I have with myself. This chapter will show you that, in fact, it is *your* words that will either help or hinder you, including in your weight and health journey.

If you use negative language, you could develop self-limiting beliefs, which will hold you back and prevent you from achieving your goals. The good news is, since these are your words, you have the power to change them. Once you have read this chapter and you start to speak the language of success, your words will change your beliefs. These new beliefs will propel you towards all the weight loss and great health that you seek.

The power of 'possible'

There is a lecture theatre at Imperial College – the Sir Roger Bannister Lecture Theatre – that I particularly enjoy teaching in because every time I do, a stopwatch displayed in a small glass cabinet catches my eye. The story of Roger Bannister and the stopwatch is the story of one of the most iconic sporting events of the twentieth century. Its message tells us everything we need to know about the word 'possible' when it comes to achieving the things we want. From weight loss to diabetes reversal, from a promotion at work to fulfilling a long-held dream, when you believe that these things are 'possible' your chance of success will sky-rocket.

In 1954, Roger Bannister, then a medical student at our hospital, had a goal: to be the first person to run a mile in under four minutes. This was the so-called 'Dream Mile', which had not yet been achieved and so had become the stuff of running legend. 'Everyone used to think it was quite impossible and beyond the reach of any runner . . .' Roger Bannister later recalled. 'But as a medical student . . . I knew this could not be true.'

On 6 May 1954, at the Oxford University racetrack, Bannister ran a mile in 3 minutes 59.4 seconds. 'The stopwatches held the answer . . . We had done it . . . !' Roger Bannister's four-minute mile is widely considered one of the greatest sporting achievements of all time.

How did Roger Bannister break the Dream Mile? This is where Bannister differed from all the other runners before him who had tried – and failed. 'Was it possible for a man to run a mile in four minutes? To me the answer was obvious. "Of course . . ."' Rather than being 'impossible', Roger Bannister had told himself a four-minute mile was 'possible'.

What came next is probably the most important part of the story. Just forty-six days later, a second runner, John Landy, not only broke the four-minute mile but ran it 1.4 seconds faster than Bannister. This is exactly what Bannister had predicted: 'It was only a question of time before [another runner] broke the barrier too . . . We had proved in Oxford that the four-minute mile was possible.'

Until 6 May 1954, no runner had been able to run a mile in four minutes. Yet since Bannister, more than two thousand runners have done so. Nothing had changed physically; what changed was the other runners' language – they now told themselves that a four-minute mile was possible. Bannister had known this all along: 'I always knew that it could not be a purely physical barrier – it had to be a psychological one.'

Roger Bannister had freed himself and the other runners from self-limiting language. He had made the 'impossible' possible.

Your brain's gatekeeper

I'm telling you this not just because it is a good story about a celebrated alumnus of my institution, but because the lessons about language are important for your Programme success.

Listening to my patients has taught me to be attuned to language. When they tell me their stories, time and again I hear the same eight words, 'It is impossible for me to lose weight.' If you are currently using these words, and in particular the word 'impossible', you are trapping yourself in the same self-limiting language as the other runners and it will prove 'impossible' for you to lose weight.

Let's explore the neuroscience behind this.

The world is too complex for your brain to let in all the external information that is constantly jostling for your attention. If it did, your senses would quickly become overwhelmed. So, your brain has a gatekeeper: a network of cells converging in a part of your brain called the thalamus that controls whether the information around you – the things you see and hear – is let in.

If information is relevant to you – to your views, beliefs, values and goals – then your gatekeeper will selectively open the gate, allowing that information to reach your conscious awareness. How does your gatekeeper know what's important to you? Because its brain cell networks are tuned into both your conscious and unconscious brain and the words you use in your internal conversations.

If you use words like, 'It is impossible for me to lose weight', your gatekeeper will selectively open the gate to information that validates this, strengthening your 'impossible' belief. So one week you weigh yourself and the scales haven't moved, you pay attention to this because it confirms that it is 'impossible' for you to lose weight. In turn, this will impact on your decision-making; for example, you will return to eating in a way that stalls your weight loss, which further confirms your self-limiting language. You can now see how your words affect your behaviour, and your behaviour governs your outcomes.

When you change your language – just as the runners after Roger Bannister did – so that you now talk about your goals being 'possible', your gatekeeper will selectively let in information that confirms this. Being open to this information – 'It is possible for me to lose weight' – will have a positive effect on your decision-making and behaviour, such as choosing to read this book and following the Programme.

> 'Your words become your actions; your
> actions become your habits . . .'

When you repeatedly carry out your new 'possible' behaviours, over time something magical happens: those behaviours start to become automatic; they turn into effortless, instinctive habits.

Habits are simply behaviours that you have learnt to carry out in response to a particular trigger. We are familiar with the habits of our daily routine, like taking a shower when the alarm goes off or walking into the kitchen and boiling the kettle. With the Programme, your new habits might include walking up an escalator rather than standing or filling your basket with fresh, healthy produce when you walk down the fruit and vegetable aisle at the supermarket.

Over time, these habits become hardwired, by changing

the connections in a part of your brain called the basal ganglia. Your habits now flow with an automatic fluidity so that once triggered (getting on the escalator, being in the fruit and veg aisle) the resulting action (walking up, buying healthy food) then becomes an instinctive, natural behaviour, which proceeds without conscious effort – no willpower required.

The science of habits and the rewiring of the basal ganglia is relatively new, but it was perhaps something that Mahatma Gandhi instinctively understood when he said, 'Your words become your actions; your actions become your habits; your habits become your values; your values become your destiny.'

The science of negative self-talk

Language is not just a way to consciously communicate information. Certain words – and here we will focus on negative, self-critical words like 'lazy/greedy/big' – will elicit a fear response in a part of your brain called your amygdala. Your amygdala responds to perceived danger – in this case your negative words – by immediately changing your body's chemistry.

Cortisol, the 'stress hormone', floods the system, which can drive weight gain, amongst other effects. The brain's 'fight-or-flight' adrenaline response is activated, making you 'wired' and hyper-vigilant to possible threats. You feel nervous, worried and uncomfortable. In this state, your gatekeeper preferentially lets in information that confirms the existence of danger and problems, which can fuel a cycle of further negative thoughts.

When you feel this way, plans to go for a swim or make a healthy Programme dinner can feel too difficult, even impossible. There's a real wisdom – now backed up by the science – that criticism withers and praise builds you up.

Since the perceived threat triggering your brain's danger response has come from your negative words, the solution – choosing new, positive words – is fully in your control. As you read on you will begin to build up a new phrase book full of the words that will take you to the weight-loss success that you deserve.

Smile and the world smiles with you

You will find, as many of my patients have, that when you change your language, using more positive and uplifting words, this will spill over into your conversations with other people. When you talk in a more upbeat way, it lifts the mood. There will be more happiness and eye contact – there's great wisdom in the saying: 'Smile and the whole world smiles with you.' We humans are social creatures and a positive inter-action like this creates feelings of connection and bonding through the brain hormone oxytocin. Oxytocin also reduces fear generation in the amygdala, lowering cortisol and damp-ening down the adrenaline-driven fight-or-flight response.

It's OK not to be OK

There is one exception to using your new positive language – it's OK not to be OK. Reframing your language is not about putting on a front or pretending that everything is awesome when in fact your mood is low or you feel anxious or unwell. In this situation, choosing to ask for help from a trusted other or healthcare professional is the right solution.

Rather, your success language is for when everything is fine or more than fine. It's at these times that all the benefits of your new way of speaking will shine through.

Becoming a contentment super-spreader

The powerful ripple effect of how we speak to other people is expressed in science as Social Contagion Theory. Happiness, like infectious diseases, spreads through your social network to your friends, family, colleagues and so on. Every time you have a positive contact with someone, the probability of your becoming contented increases. If you choose to use your uplifting language to become a contentment super-spreader, people will respond positively to you and want to be in your company. This will make you feel good and your confidence will soar.

Roger Bannister said of his attempt on the 'Dream Mile': 'We can allow ourselves to be blown along like leaves in a storm, or we can try to take action.' With these words in mind, it's time to consider whether to take action and to start speaking a new language of success using these choices.

CHOICES

Choice 1: Ditch the negative words

When you speak this new language, you will become increasingly attuned to the power of words. It's not just the word 'impossible'. As you explore your current language, you might come across other self-limiting words. These might be wrapped up in statements that you tell yourself are 'jokes' about being 'old' or 'clumsy', 'slow' or 'big'. In fact, you now know that these 'jokes' give you the message, 'This is who I am', and your brain will pay attention to and prioritize information that confirms this, which will create barriers to you achieving the outcomes you seek.

Even if you are not using such obviously self-critical words, you might also want to listen out for subtler negative self-talk. The word 'just' is an example of this. For instance, when someone asks what you do, do you answer, 'I'm just a . . .'? Before learning the new Programme language, many of my patients would answer in this way: 'I'm just a stay-at-home-mum', or 'I just work part-time.' That little word 'just' in fact packs a big punch because it is deeply undermining. Instead, you could choose language that implies pride in what you do: 'I am a . . .'

'I hope' is another phrase to watch out for. 'I hope' is a doubt statement that implies the outcome you seek is not within your control. If Roger Bannister had said, 'I hope I can run a four-minute mile', he would have diminished his chance of success. Instead, you can change 'I hope I can lose weight' to words packed full of certainty like, 'I will lose weight' or 'I am going to lose weight.'

Lastly, there are two words that might be holding you back from losing weight and reclaiming your health: 'Yes, but . . .' If you tune into your language, you could find you are using, 'Yes, but . . .' as a reason not to take action. For example, with regards to the Eating Window, you might be saying:

'Yes, but . . . my family like to eat late', or 'Yes, but . . . my schedule is too unpredictable to have Eating Window timings.'

'Yes, but . . .' is a way of deflecting possible solutions to issues like weight loss. By discarding, 'Yes, but . . .' you will instead be open to using your Programme tools to lose weight and feel good.

Choice 2: Embrace the three Cs

The three Cs are very powerful words in your Programme dictionary: Choice, Choose, Choosing.

The three Cs invariably come up when we discuss food options in the Programme for the first time. My patients, who haven't yet learnt the new language, will ask, 'Am I allowed to eat . . . ?' The answer is – of course! My patients are allowed to eat everything because this Programme is not about being told what to do. Like you, my patients are adults who can live their life in any way that they choose. It's therefore not for me or for anybody else to say, 'This is allowed and this isn't allowed.' They, and you, do not need permission. Instead, this is where the three Cs come in.

To choose to do something is to tell yourself, 'I like this, I want to do this, I am pleased with this action or behaviour.' Contrast, 'I am not allowed to eat biscuits', with 'I am choosing not to eat biscuits.' In the first statement you are a passive participant who is asking somebody else to take responsibility. In the second 'choosing' statement, it is you that is fully in control.

Describing your Programme tools in terms of Choice, Choose, Choosing will make it even more likely that you will enjoy and continue to use them. The three Cs make it clear that using your tools is a positive decision and you are in charge.

Choice 3: Choose to practise your new language of success

If you have learnt a new language before, you'll remember that practice makes perfect and that you become increasingly fluent the more you speak the language. It's the same with reframing your language; the more you practise your new Programme language, the more you will find yourself speaking in a way that is consistent with the outcomes you want.

So instead of saying, 'I can't eat snacks in the evening', you can say, 'I like how in control I feel with my Eating Window.' Rather than thinking about exercise and saying to yourself, 'What a hassle, I can't be bothered', you can change your language and tell yourself, 'I like going for my walk because I feel so good afterwards.'

Elite athletes know that no matter how fit and talented they are, success is all about the way in which they choose to talk to themselves. So instead of putting themselves down, they consistently use words to hardwire the habits of success.

You can see this in the language of our most celebrated athletes. Let's take the basketball player Michael 'Air' Jordan, one of the greatest sports stars of all time. It is known that Jordan never allowed himself to think about failure. Instead, he would say, 'Why would I think about missing a shot I haven't taken yet?'

If, like Michael Jordan, you want to give yourself the best chance of success, you can choose not to talk about results that you don't want – 'Why would I think about missing a shot I haven't taken yet?' – and instead fill your language with all of the outcomes that you seek.

This is what my patient Meriem did, whose heartfelt words open this chapter. At first, Meriem wasn't sure that she could speak in this new positive language but, encouraged by others in her Programme group, Meriem found that this way of speaking was to prove empowering – losing 3 stone 7lb (22kg) and reversing her diabetes. 'We have come a long and rich way from despair to enlightenment,' Meriem said, 'from the impossible to the possible.'

You might be worried, like Meriem was initially, that you can't tap into these techniques because you are different from people like Roger Bannister or Michael Jordan. In fact, we are all the same and we can all choose to use the language of success. As Bannister himself said, 'However ordinary each of us may seem, we are all in some way special and can do things that are extraordinary, perhaps until then even thought impossible.'

CHAPTER 11

Goals

**'Good morning Dr Saira, good news! My
order arrived today . . . I am absolutely over
the moon. Hit my weight-loss goal!'
Elaine, lost 3 stone 9lb (23kg)**

Whatever you want to achieve in life, your goals are your
internal compass guiding you to the outcomes you seek. This
chapter is about setting your goals using a powerfully effective system that will clearly define what you want and how
you are going to get there. By using these techniques, just
as my very successful patients have done, you will be giving
yourself the best possible advantage for achieving your
weight-loss goals.

What do you want?
Scroll the store, add to basket

The first step for goal setting is to know, with absolute precision, what you want. You might think the answer is obvious:
'I want to lose weight', but this isn't specific enough. Instead,

your success will flow from stating very precisely what your goals are.

In our Programme groups, to help my patients decide *exactly* what they want, we imagine every possible goal being available on a vast online store ('MyProgrammeGoals.com'!). Every goal listed on the site is available to you too, but there are so many different goals to choose from that you need to be very specific about what you want. Otherwise you might end up getting waylaid by something else and giving up on your original search or even buying the wrong thing altogether.

Answering these questions will help you to choose a realistic weight-loss goal that fits with your biology and your objectives:

1. **What's my build?**
   There are three factors you can take into account here – your height and shoe size, as well as your wrist size – which will give you a good idea about the size of your skeleton. The gauge is when you grip your wrist bones with the thumb and forefinger of the opposite hand – if your thumb and forefinger overlap you are likely to have a small frame, if they touch you have a medium build and if they don't meet you are well-built. Taken together with your shoe size and height, you can work out your overall build, which you can use as a guide for choosing your goal weight.

2.   **What's the lowest weight I've been as an adult?**
     This question is followed up with:
     Was it hard or easy to maintain that weight?
     Your body has a weight set-point controlled by your
     brain's weight-control centre (the hypothalamus).
     If you go lower than your weight set-point through
     intensive restrictive dieting, the hypothalamus will try
     to pull your weight back up to its natural set-point
     where it feels comfortable. This means a weight goal
     that's too low is difficult to maintain because you will
     be fighting your biology.

3.   **What weight has best suited me?**
     This is what I call 'my happy weight'. At this weight,
     life felt good and you had an inner sense of ease.
     Your clothes were comfortable and you felt energetic.
     If you have developed health issues such as diabetes
     because of your weight, then it's also helpful to
     consider the weight threshold that you crossed when
     you developed these conditions.

4.   **What's important to me?**
     When you are clear about *why* your weight-loss
     goal is important, you are more likely to achieve
     it because we commit more strongly to goals
     we consider valuable. You will have joined the
     Programme because you want to lose weight, but
     the real Programme magic is what that weight-loss
     goal means in your everyday life or, put another

way, why being that particular weight is meaningful to you. For example, getting to a goal might be associated with health improvements, like coming off medications. Or reaching your goal weight might mean wearing different sorts of clothes (new clothes tend to be a side-effect of the Programme).

You have now chosen your specific goal from our online store and you can click *Add to basket*. But hold off placing your order for a moment because if you include some extra delivery instructions, then you will significantly increase the chances of your order being fulfilled.

Your extra delivery instructions: making your goals happen

Now that you have identified *what* you want and *why*, the next step is to figure out the *how* – which Programme tools am I going to use to achieve my goal?

Let's say you have identified that avoiding ultra-processed foods is key to your weight-loss goal, then your tool might be taking a Programme-food packed lunch to work. This keeps you fully in control of your food choices and protected from the tricks of the food industry.

You can give yourself the best chance of consistently using your chosen tool by making a definite plan about the *when*, *where* and *how* of incorporating that Programme tool into your everyday life.

For example: 'When my alarm goes off at 7am (that's the

when), I'll go into the kitchen (that's the *where*) to make myself a packed lunch using ingredients from the fridge and store cupboard (that's the *how*).'

This strategic, planned approach is especially powerful when combined with a 'nudge' that prompts you to carry out the action – for example, putting your lunchbox on the kitchen counter every night so that it is ready and waiting for you in the morning. The evidence shows that the easier we make an action, the more likely it is to happen.

You are now certain about *what* you want and *why* and *how* you will make sure your order will be delivered. Now for the exciting part – it's time to click *Place my order*.

See your success

Once you have placed your order and are working towards your goal, there's another technique called visualization – 'seeing' your goal in your mind's eye or imagination – that increases the probability of achieving it. For example, you might choose to 'see' your goal weight when you stand on the scales or 'watch' yourself buying new clothes.

When you visualize an action, this activates (or 'lights up') the same parts of your brain that you use when you actually perform the action in real life. Over time, a new pathway is created in your brain as groups of brain cells learn to work together in order to perform the action – even though you are just imagining it! This is known as Motor Imagery Practice, which you can think of as a sort of brain training. Visualization is particularly powerful when it comes to weight loss. In a randomized controlled trial that compared visualization to a behaviour change technique, after a year the visualization group had lost almost ten times more weight (1 stone/6.44kg) than the behaviour change group, who had lost less than a kilogram (1.5lb/0.67kg).

You are now equipped with your Programme goal-setting know-how, including how 'seeing' your success will power-charge your progress. The choices you are going to read about will now frame these techniques in a practical guide to achieving your goals – order fulfilled!

CHOICES

Choice 1: Be specific

Step one is choosing exactly *what* you want and *why* you want it. This is most effective when you are specific:

'I want . . .'
'This is important to me because . . .'

For example, 'I want to lose 2 stone (13kg). This is important to me because I want to enjoy running around with my children.'

If your overall goal feels like too much to do at once, then you can break it down into mini-goals using the same principles:

'I want to lose a stone (6.5 kg) to feel more
energetic when we go to the park. Once I've done
this, I want to lose another stone (6.5 kg) so that
I am fit enough to play football with my girls.'

You can also now join the dots between your actions (the
Programme tools you will use) and the outcomes you want:

'I will use . . . to achieve . . .'

For example, 'I will close my Eating Window at 7pm to put
myself in control of late-night snacking.'

Next, you can choose to make a definite plan about *when*,
where and *how* you will implement these intentions.

For example:

When	Where	How
In the evening, at 7pm	. . . in the kitchen	. . . I will finish my dinner and then close my Eating Window

Choice 2: Track your progress

Once you have defined your goals, you can now decide how
to track your progress. For some people this will mean weighing themselves, but the scales aren't for everyone. Instead,
other people like to monitor their progress by how their
clothes fit. Or, if you have health conditions related to your

weight, you can also keep an eye on how these improve over time. For example, my patients with diabetes know they are on track when they see their home blood-sugar checks start to run at normal.

Alternatively, you can monitor your progress by how you feel. This is perhaps the most important feedback of all. If you feel good and strong, then it's likely that all is going well. In our Programme research study, we compared our participants' wellbeing at the start and then again six months into the Programme. We measured many elements of wellbeing – including general health, energy and emotional wellbeing – and all had significantly improved during the Programme. This formal assessment of wellbeing confirmed what we had already observed – the surge in happiness and positivity in our group, as my patients clocked up their successes and achieved their goals. You can use these questions, adapted from those we used in our research study, as a barometer to judge your own wellbeing:

- How physically fit am I feeling; for example, does climbing stairs now feel more comfortable?
- Do I usually have enough energy to get me through the day?
- Do I find it easier to get things done and to take part in things?
- Does socializing feel more enjoyable?
- Do I generally feel an inner sense of contentment?

<u>Making the scales work for you</u>

Body weight can naturally fluctuate from day to day; for example, after eating a salty meal or for some women their periods (menstrual cycle) can temporarily affect their weight. These small weight changes are not important to your overall direction of travel. To avoid being distracted by these minor fluctuations, it's best to weigh yourself just once a week. This will give you more accurate information about your progress towards your goal.

Choice 3: Make your success movie and choose your happy ending

In our groups, my patients structure their visualization by making a 'success movie' that they 'watch' in their heads. The content of the movie is about your goal and how it feels to achieve it. Importantly, it should have a happy ending – order fulfilled, goal achieved! So you might 'see' yourself looking fit and healthy at an upcoming family wedding or 'hear' your doctor telling you your blood tests are now normal.

You can choose to 'watch' your movie several times a day, whenever you have a moment of downtime – walking to work or waiting for the kettle to boil. The sprinter Michael Johnson describes doing just that. 'Any time I wasn't doing something that required my full attention my mind defaulted back to thinking about and visualizing races,' Johnson said. 'I would automatically imagine the gun going off . . . I could go inside my own mind . . . I focused on running a perfect race in my head.' Johnson won thirteen Olympic and World Championship gold medals and was called the 'Fastest Man in the World'. Just like Michael Johnson, you too can run a perfect Programme race in your head, except your gold medal is achieving your weight-loss goal.

You are now ready to set up your goals to maximize your chances of success by:

- Being specific about what you want
- Choosing the Programme tools that will get you there
- Visualizing your goal achieved

These are the techniques my patients used to achieve their outstanding weight-loss results. Like Elaine, who lost 3 stone 9lb (23kg) and whose words open this chapter: 'My order arrived today . . . I am absolutely over the moon. Hit my weight-loss goal!' After many years of resolutions and then trying again, by setting her goals the Programme way, Elaine's order had been delivered – she had achieved her goal.

CHAPTER 12

Brain gains

**'The session on gain was amazing and it
was really pertinent. I feel liberated having
gone through a process of understanding
myself. The work is now to discard old beliefs
and sew in new beliefs and behaviours.'**
Vineet, lost 1 stone 8lb (10kg)

If you have ever lost weight only to then regain it, or if
you find yourself not using your Programme tools, such as
food choices and exercise, please be kind to yourself. You
are not 'weak-willed' or any other discouraging words you
might have used. Instead, this could be happening because
of programming in a part of your brain that has learnt that
these behaviours have a gain – meaning a benefit – for you.
This part of your brain, called the limbic system, is not
trying to trip you up. In fact, it's quite the reverse. Your
brain is acting as your guardian because the gain (benefit) –
as far as the limbic system is concerned – is about keeping
you safe.

In this chapter we'll explore why your limbic system might have learnt that being a certain weight keeps you safe. And we will also look at how you can use another part of your brain to override these limbic safety behaviours and instead generate actions that are consistent with your weight-loss goals.

Situation: response

Through millions of years of evolution we have developed a particularly high-tech part of the brain called the prefrontal cortex (the bit of your brain behind your forehead). It is the prefrontal cortex that contains many of our thinking abilities, such as memory, logic, self-control and emotional processing – so we'll call it the Thinking Brain.

Compared to the 250-million-year-old Ancient Brain (limbic system), the Thinking Brain is an evolutionary newcomer of only about two to three million years old. Although we now have a state-of-the-art 'Thinking Brain', as we evolved we didn't discard our Ancient Brain, which we had used for the millions of years before our Thinking Brain developed.

One of the reasons we have held on to our Ancient Brain is that it remains useful to us today. Through a combination of learning from our life experiences as well as inbuilt programming, from an early age our Ancient Brain develops a behavioural repertoire that keeps us safe. This allows the Ancient Brain (and, in particular, the amygdala, which we met in Chapter 10), to react immediately when it perceives a threat, without the need for conscious thought. This automatic response to danger gives us a survival advantage. If we see a sabre-toothed tiger, we don't have time to think things through or consider all the options, we need to generate a split-second behaviour – RUN!

Over the years, you will also have learnt whether weight loss is advantageous or could in fact be seen as 'unsafe' for some reason. If losing weight is perceived as a threat by your Ancient Brain, it can sometimes default to safety behaviours that it has learnt are in your best interests – even if those actions aren't in keeping with your weight-loss goals.

Everyday Gains

In my clinical experience, there are a number of reasons why the Ancient Brain might perceive weight loss as threatening. The Everyday Gains listed below reflect many years of caring for people with weight issues and hundreds of conversations with my patients. These Everyday Gains are discussed at our group sessions and you too can consider if any of these examples are relevant to your own situation:

1. **Partner relations**

    'When I lose weight this upsets the relationship applecart with my partner. My new way of eating and lifestyle changes cause tensions between us. It's safer to go back to the old ways to restore the status quo.'

Although weight loss can be very positive for a couple, for some people it can cause a strain by changing the relationship's dynamics. When someone loses weight, they might become more confident, dress differently, socialize more or find a new job.

2. Friendship dynamics

'My changes make other people uncomfortable and they say things like, "You're no fun now", or "I feel like I don't know you any more." Remaining at a higher weight puts me back into my usual role and my friends continue to approve of me, which keeps me safe.'

Weight loss and making healthy choices can sometimes disrupt friendships in which you were playing a particular part (more on this in Chapter 14). If you were the person who could always be relied on to order dessert or stay up late and now you are choosing new behaviours, this forces other people to review their own choices. Your changes can make others feel unnerved – even guilty – about not taking charge of their own health or weight situation.

3. Shielding smokescreen

'Instead of pushing myself to pursue dreams or take new opportunities, I can use my weight to guard against the possibility of rejection or failure. It allows me to tell myself, "I *would* have applied for that promotion", or "I *would* have asked that person out, but I didn't because of my weight."'

4. Completely cared for

'Carrying extra weight means that I receive care, concern or attention from family, friends or health professionals, and this makes me feel safe.'

5. Protective jacket

'My Ancient Brain has conflated being a certain weight with being protected and able to stand up for myself.'

Here, weight can feel like a protective insulator. One of my patients described this feeling as like being cocooned in a warm puffer jacket. Others of my patients have wondered whether being a certain weight keeps other people at arm's length.

This is not a definitive list, but these examples demonstrate how, if losing weight could be perceived as a threat, your Ancient Brain could be generating behaviours that sabotage your weight-loss efforts.

Encouragingly, as many of my patients have done, it is possible to stop these unhelpful 'safety' behaviours and instead to generate new actions that will help you live at the weight you want to be. The choices coming up will explain how you can do this.

CHOICES

Choice 1: Press pause and use your Thinking Brain

Incoming information hits your Ancient Brain very quickly. It has to, in case you are encountering a threat to your survival – a tiger (run!), oncoming traffic (jump back on the kerb!). However, when there's no imminent danger, we can allow the Thinking Brain the time it needs to sift through and analyse the information. The Thinking Brain can then generate a response that is consistent with losing weight, which might include blocking Ancient Brain-generated behaviours.

How do these two parts of your brain work in everyday life? When you say 'no' to going out for pizza and your friends respond with, 'You're no fun any more', the 'threat' of their disapproval will quickly hit your Ancient Brain. If this is the only part of the brain you use, then you will generate a split-second response that keeps you 'safe' within the group: 'Sure, let's have pizza.'

If instead you 'press pause', you will allow the information – eating pizza – to be processed by your Thinking Brain, which draws on high-level information like your weight-loss goals to generate a response: 'I don't fancy pizza, how about we go to that great new fish restaurant?'

These situations are often predictable, so you will be in an even better position if you can use your Thinking Brain in advance to decide how to react. This will result in a calm, logical response: 'My friends' disapproval is not a threat. They're just unsettled by my new way of eating. I won't let this get in the way of my weight loss.' Here, you've used your Thinking Brain to make decisions based on what's important to you – losing weight.

Choice 2: 'What's the gain?'

Initially, at our 'Brain gains' session, some of my patients say, 'There's nothing worse for me than being overweight, there is definitely no benefit in self-sabotaging or remaining at a higher weight. I'm certain this doesn't apply to me.' That could certainly be the case and you may feel the same. But before you finalize this conclusion, perhaps allow yourself to be curious about the ideas in this chapter, which could give you a new awareness about yourself and the things that you do.

With this in mind, I ask my patients to take time to consider the following – and you can do this too:

1. Do you ask self-critical questions, like 'Why did I do that?' or 'What's wrong with me?' This could be a signpost that your Ancient Brain is driving your behaviour. You then have the option to press pause and allow your Thinking Brain to generate more logical, thoughtful behaviours that will help you to lose weight.

2. You can ask yourself, is there a reason to keep the weight on or to regain weight after losing it? Perhaps there is something about weight loss – like the disapproval of others – that makes it safer not to make changes.

3. You can review the five Everyday Gains described in this chapter to ask whether these or other Everyday Gains are impacting on your weight loss:
    •   Partner relations
    •   Friendship dynamics
    •   Shielding smokescreen
    •   Completely cared for
    •   Protective jacket

4. As you think these ideas through, you might feel some more support would be helpful. If so, following up with your GP for additional help or advice could be beneficial.

For many of my patients, like Vineet, who said at the start of the chapter, 'I feel liberated having gone through a process of understanding myself', these ideas can be a revelation. Vineet, who lost 1 stone 8lb (10kg) and came off his blood-pressure tablets, reversed his diabetes and used his new self-knowledge to review and refresh his behaviours to get the outcomes he wanted.

Using your Thinking Brain can also reduce quick-fire safety responses in other areas of your life, like the tendency to say no to opportunities. We see this in our groups when people report back good news stories like: 'I gave the keynote speech at our company conference.' 'I'm going travelling.' 'We're getting married!'

If this chapter resonates with you, I hope you can use these ideas to question any previously limiting thoughts and behaviours that had been holding back your weight loss and to develop new ways of thinking that unlock your own potential for living life to the full.

CHAPTER 13

Feelings

'Merry Christmas Doc, wishing you a
wonderful day, thank you so much for
everything you are giving me. A new life.'
Paul, lost 7 stone 2lb (45kg)

When it comes to losing weight, 'Why do I eat when I'm not hungry?' is the million-dollar question. If we only ate according to biological hunger, when the stomach's hunger signal (ghrelin) was strong, we would eat to meet the body's needs and then stop. But if there are times you find yourself eating when ghrelin is not sending a hunger text message to your brain, this chapter will help you to understand the reasons why.

We will look at your 'two brains': your Head Brain – in which sugary pick-me-up foods change your brain's chemistry and hijack control of your eating; and we'll also look at your 'other brain' – the 'brain' in your gut, which plays a fundamental role in your feelings, which in turn impact on your eating. We'll then go through practical strategies that will help you to lose weight by developing a new, easier, happier relationship with food.

Soothed with food – emotional feeding

For many of us, childhood upsets were soothed with food – a tantrum consoled with a bag of sweets, a fall from the swings made better by an ice cream. If this pattern (known as emotional feeding) sounds familiar, then although it is often done with the best of intentions, it might have taught you to respond to sadness or stress by eating.

The foods that we learn to soothe ourselves with are usually sugary and ultra-processed. They make us feel better because they elicit a rush of the brain chemical (neurotransmitter) dopamine in the brain's reward centre. This is the same dopamine pleasure rush that the brain experiences if you take drugs like cocaine or amphetamine, gamble, play video games or get 'likes' on social media. So it's understandable why we can look to foods like chocolate, ice cream and biscuits to lift our mood when we feel low or stressed.

Brain chemicals like dopamine work by attaching to receptors found on brain cells. If you think of dopamine being like a key, the receptor is the lock it fits into to open the door (produce an effect in brain cells). If we repeatedly eat these pleasure-rush foods to cheer ourselves up, the reward centre becomes bombarded with dopamine. To protect itself, the reward centre reduces the availability of receptors for dopamine to attach to. This is like removing the locks on a door to prevent the door being opened, even though keys (dopamine) are available.

Now, when we eat chocolate, ice cream and biscuits, without enough receptors available, the dopamine rush is diminished – the reward-centre pleasure door can't be opened. So we end up eating more and more of these sugary, processed foods, chasing that elusive 'first-hit' feeling in a biological process known as 'tolerance'.

This is where the Programme helps. As you read on, we will explore ways to look after yourself when you're feeling down or stressed that don't involve food, but instead give your mind the care and nurture that it needs.

Gut feelings

Aside from the brain in your head, you have another brain – a brain in your gut, known as the enteric nervous system (your Gut Brain), which contains more nerve cells than your spinal cord.

Your Gut Brain uses the same neurotransmitters (chemical signals) as your Head Brain, including the mood-boosting 'happy hormone' serotonin. In fact, more than 90 per cent of your body's serotonin is made in your gut and scientists are now researching whether anti-depressants like Prozac, which increase serotonin levels, are working in the gut and even on the gut bacteria.

The presence of a brain in the gut explains why the language we use to describe our emotions is often tied up with food and eating. Difficult experiences are 'gut-wrenching'. An upsetting situation makes us feel 'sick to the stomach'. When faced with an important decision, we take the time to 'digest' the information, while other times we just trust our 'gut instincts'. When we feel overwhelmed, we might say, 'I have too much on my plate.' These are your 'gut feelings', which flow between your Gut Brain and your Head Brain through the vagus nerve, which acts like a telephone cable, transmitting information between the two.

Once you understand the Gut Brain–Head Brain connection, you can see why feelings can be physically experienced in the gut. The knot in your stomach when you are upset, the butterflies when you are excited, having an 'upset' tummy when you are sad or unhappy. Similarly, being low, bored or lonely can be physically experienced in the gut as a feeling of emptiness – being 'drained' or even 'gutted'. A common response to these feelings is to try to 'fill up' the emptiness with food even though you aren't hungry.

You can now see how your two brains might be contributing to eating when you are not physically hungry. Eating sugary foods when you're stressed generates a dopamine high in your Head Brain, that you need to eat more pleasure-rush foods to sustain. And if your Gut Brain feels emotionally empty, you might try to make that emptiness go away by filling up with food.

If one or both of these situations resonates with you, please don't worry. Many of my patients also felt this way until they started to use the practical advice that you are going to read about to deal with stress and to get full without using food.

CHOICES

Choice 1: Consider whether there are some foods that will never work for you

Let's start with your Head Brain. Now that you know the neuroscience you'll understand why there could be some foods, such as ice cream and biscuits, that will never work for you. Instead, you might conclude, like many of my patients have, that you will only get in control of these sugary, ultra-processed foods by cutting them out completely. After a period of time, whenever we quit a dopamine-generating substance or behaviour – from sugary food to cocaine, to gambling and social media – the reward centre no longer pushes you to trigger the next dopamine hit and you will become a person who *used* to eat these foods.

You will find that by taking out a few foods that don't work with your brain's chemistry, you will be getting back control of your eating. This is what we found in our Programme research study – people whose eating had been out of control for many years were now enjoying a much easier relationship with food in which they controlled their eating, rather than the other way around.

Choice 2: How to turn your back on dopamine-rush foods

Once you are up and running, shunning these foods will become a natural part of your eating routine. However, when you first quit these foods, staying on track will require some know-how. Over the years, my patients have used some or all of these strategies, and I hope you find these ideas helpful too:

- Don't keep foods in the house that bombard your reward centre. At the end of a long or difficult day, if there are no biscuits in the cupboard or ice cream in the freezer, it is far easier to not eat them.
- If you used to snack on sugary foods, make sure Programme snacks like fruit, nuts and seeds, crudités, olives and cheese are easily available to you at home, as well as carrying them in your bag and keeping them at work.
- Make sure you are eating enough Programme foods to keep your ghrelin hunger signal turned down. Otherwise, feeling hungry will make these sugary foods more appealing when you see chocolate displayed at the checkout or are offered biscuits in a meeting.
- Get enough sleep! As we saw in Chapter 6, when sleep has turned down the ghrelin hunger signal and your mind is refreshed and sharp, it is far easier to steer clear of the foods you used to eat to keep yourself going.
- Rather than relying on certain foods to manage stress, let the Programme be your stress-reduction technique – the next choice will show you how.

Choice 3: Choose the Programme as your stress-reduction technique

Since stress-eating is common, you might be surprised that there is not a chapter or choice called 'Stress Reduction'. This is deliberate. In the Programme, we've explored a range of 'stress-reduction' techniques, like mindfulness, gratitude practices, journalling and breathing exercises. All of these are good ways to reduce stress, but no single stress-reduction method resonated sufficiently strongly with the majority of my patients, who also taught me this:

> The Programme is a stress-reduction technique

This is because the Programme gives you tools to care for and nurture yourself, so you are better able to work through a stressful situation:

- You are off the blood-sugar rollercoaster and have lost the daily irritability and fatigue that comes from blood sugar crashes.
- You have lost weight and your confidence has increased.
- You are getting enough sleep so your mood is brighter, you are energized and your thoughts are clear and organized.

- You choose not to be still and instead you keep moving, creating a sense of inner calm – that mind first aid from Chapter 5.

Yes, there will always be stress in life – but rather than turning to food, you are now mentally and physically in the best possible position to weather the storm until it eventually clears.

Choice 4: Fill up with something more satisfying than food

The next time you feel Gut Brain emptiness, before trying to fill it up with food, you can instead ask yourself, 'How can I fill myself up without eating?' The answer might be calling someone who always makes you feel good (who fills you up), going for a walk or hugging your kids. All of these activities will fill up your emotional hunger in a way that food never could.

My patient Paul, whose words open this chapter, chose to fill up on cycling and would often share his daily progress with me: '19 March – 21.7 miles; 20 March – 10.3 miles; Yesterday – 33.1 miles.' By boosting his endorphins (feel-good hormones), cycling filled Paul up and in the process he lost 7 stone 2lb (45 kg) and reversed his type 2 diabetes.

If you identify a specific situation or person that makes you feel empty – collectively called 'Drainers' – you can think about stopping or minimizing your exposure to them. You are not making an inherent judgment about the Drainer,

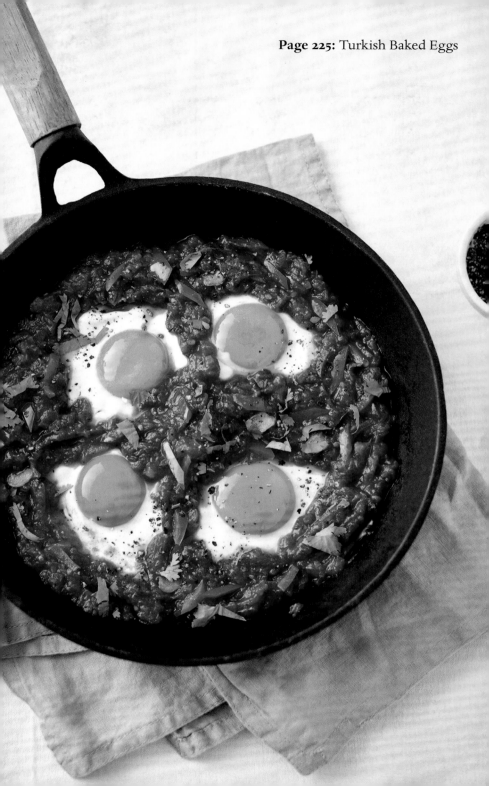

Page 225: Turkish Baked Eggs

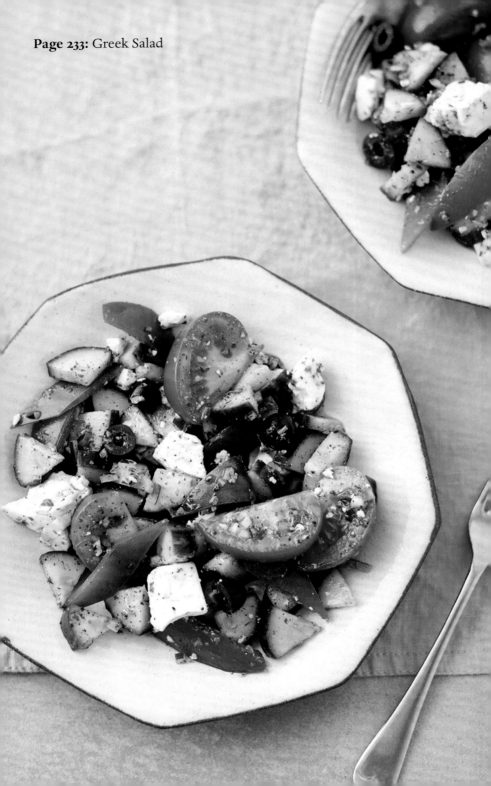

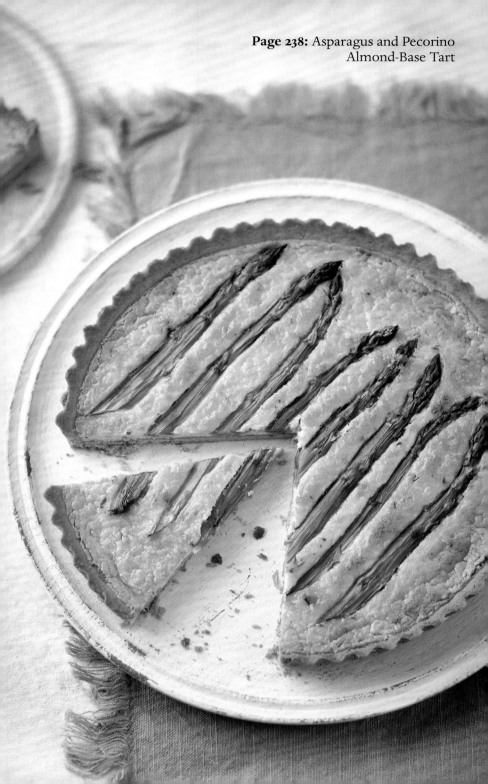

Page 238: Asparagus and Pecorino
Almond-Base Tart

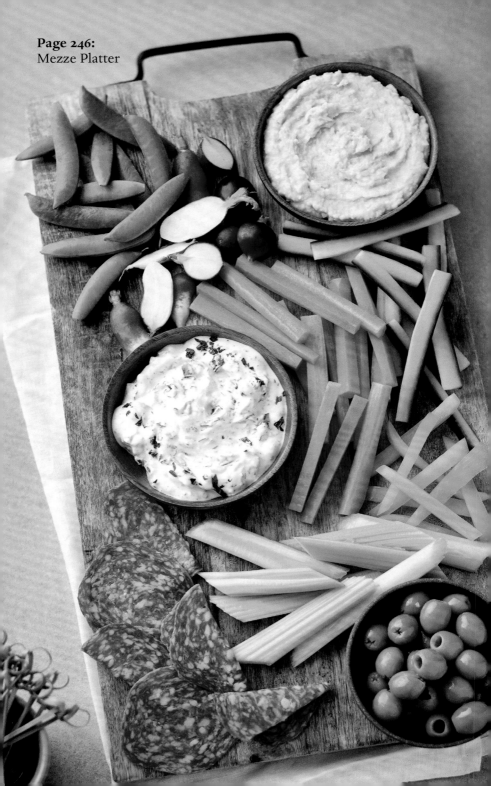

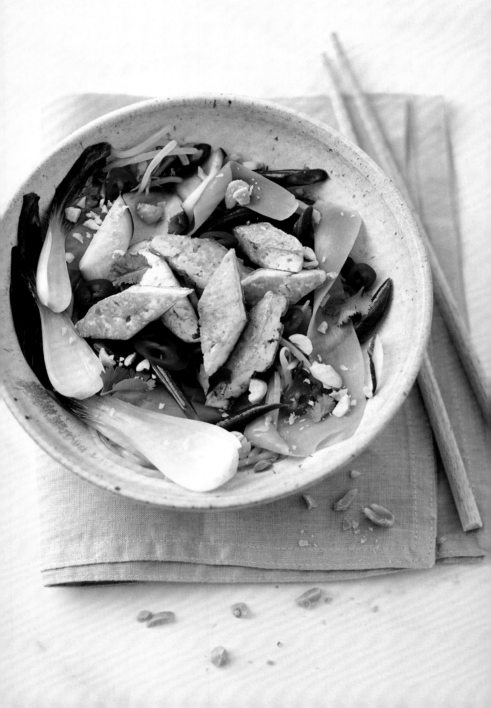

Page 254: Tofu and Mixed Vegetable Stir-fry

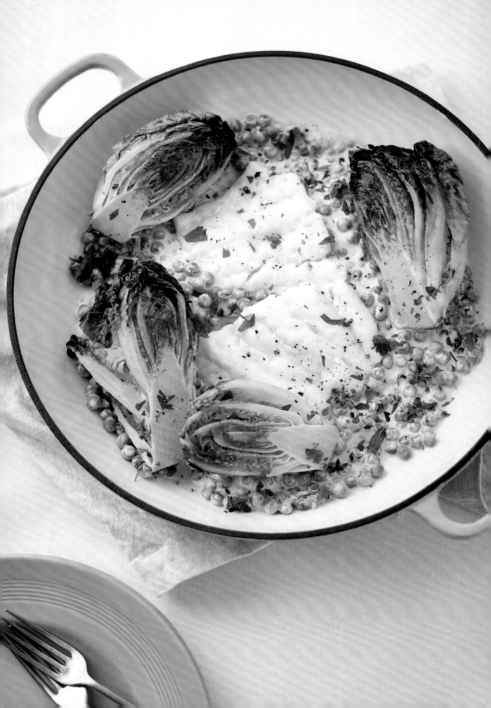

Page 267: Braised Cod with Lettuce, Peas and Crème Fraîche

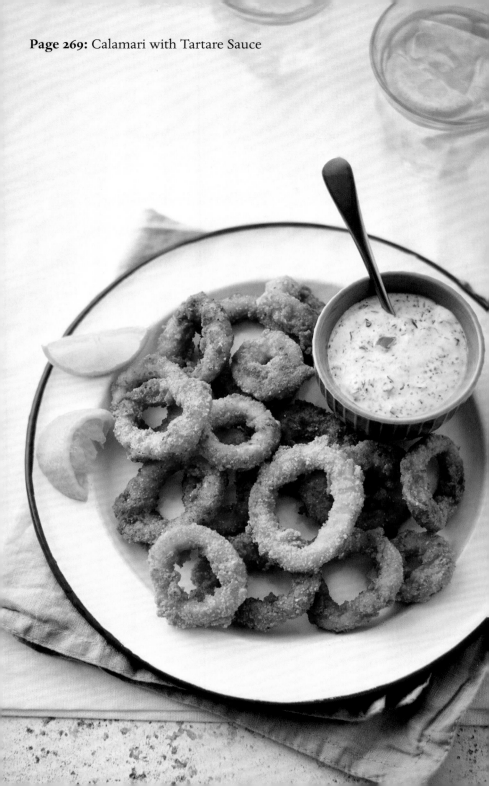

Page 269: Calamari with Tartare Sauce

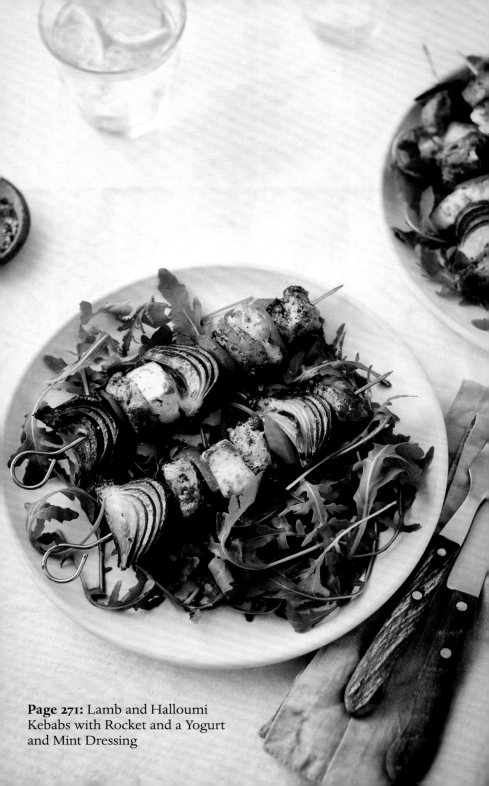

Page 271: Lamb and Halloumi Kebabs with Rocket and a Yogurt and Mint Dressing

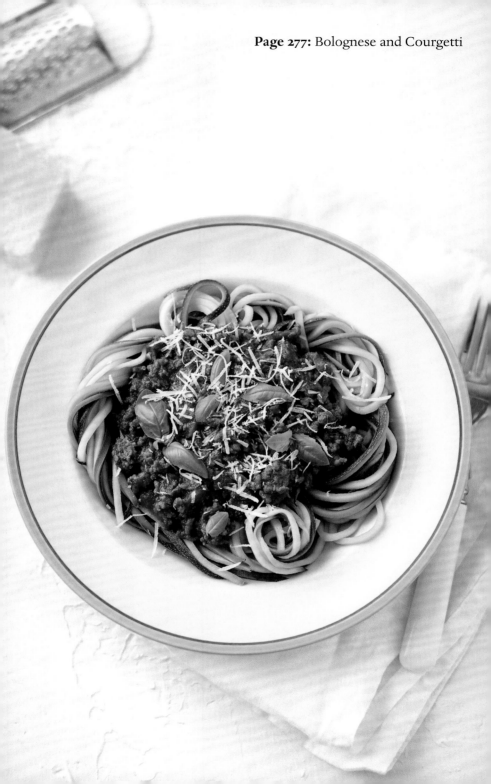

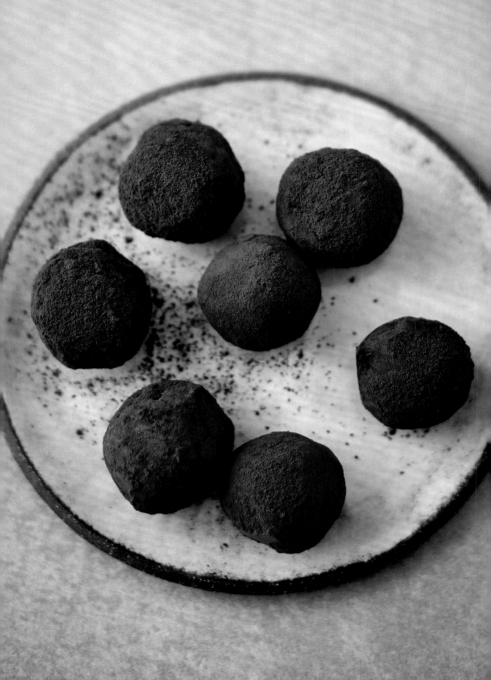

Page 279: Dark Chocolate Truffles

lean people. You can then decide whether you want to use them too.

SECRETS

Secret 1: 'Naturally' lean people eat when they are hungry and stop when they are full

'Naturally' lean people are attuned to their hunger–fullness signalling system. They eat when their ghrelin hunger signal is strong and they stop when their fullness text messages tell them to, even if it means leaving food on their plate. The Programme will reboot your hunger–fullness signalling system, but at first listening in to your body's needs will require some deliberate effort and concentration. Keep going, because soon your body's messages will be coming through loud and clear. Then – like a 'naturally' lean person – you will know with absolute certainty when to eat and when to stop.

Secret 2: 'Naturally' lean people eat slowly

'Naturally' lean people eat slowly, which strengthens their fullness hormone messages. You might have noticed that they take smaller bites, they chew their food thoroughly and they pause between mouthfuls.

You can choose to eat slowly too, maximizing your fullness signalling. And unlike restrictive diets, the Programme is a celebration of food and eating. So when you slow down and use your senses to experience every bite, your eating will be even more enjoyable.

Secret 3: 'Naturally' lean people are OK with occasionally being hungry

'Naturally' lean people are sometimes hungry when it's not convenient to eat or the right food isn't available. In these situations, rather than finding a way to eat immediately, 'naturally' lean people will 'sit with' their hunger for a short period. You can choose to do this too. It's important to emphasize that the Programme is *not* about restricting food or *deliberately* going hungry. Rather, if there are times when you can't eat Programme food straight away, it's better to tap into your body's fuel tanks than to eat off-Programme food just to instantly make the hunger go away.

For example, if you feel hungry on your evening commute, instead of buying whatever's available to immediately turn off your hunger, it's better to wait a short time and eat your delicious Programme food when you get home. The game-changer here is that unlike restrictive diets that cannot satisfy hunger, when it next becomes convenient to eat, your Programme food will fill you up. I hope this helps you to re-frame hunger from something that *always* requires urgent attention to simply – like all of your body's messages – being a guide that is on your side.

Secret 4: 'Naturally' lean people know it's NEAT to keep moving

This secret takes us back to NEAT – non-exercise activity thermogenesis – that we looked at in Chapter 5. NEAT encompasses all our little moments of movement outside of formal exercise, like standing on public transport or taking the stairs. Studies consistently show an association between high NEAT levels and a healthy body weight. There are some suggestions on pages 86–7 for building NEAT into your day – now that you know this NEAT secret of 'naturally' lean people, you can choose to use it too.

Secret 5: Some 'naturally' lean people are unhealthy

Just because someone looks lean, it doesn't mean they're healthy. It's important to mention this, because sometimes at our sessions my patients mention a 'naturally' lean person they know who eats ultra-processed food or does no exercise, yet is not overweight. The missing piece of information here is – this person may be lean, but are they healthy?

There is a group of people known as TOFI – thin-on-the-outside-fat-on-the-inside. TOFI is the scientific description of someone who appears to be thin because they have little fat under their skin (the sort of fat that changes our body size). However, what they do have is unseen internal fat (called visceral fat), which accumulates in the abdomen and infiltrates organs such as the liver. Visceral fat is associated with insulin resistance and illnesses like diabetes and high blood pressure.

So this secret comes with a buyer-beware warning – we want to be in on the secrets of *healthy* lean people. If someone is not overweight but appears to be making unhealthy lifestyle choices, this is not somebody we want to learn from. Unfortunately, they might have hidden visceral fat – a concealed metabolic time-bomb – despite being thin on the outside and appearing to be 'naturally' lean.

Secret 6: 'Naturally' lean people don't have a dieter's catastrophizing mindset

Sometimes, despite being tuned into their biology, 'naturally' lean people eat too much or eat sugary food because they are bored. The difference is that they then move on with their day, whereas some of my patients used to catastrophize a similar misstep. One glitch would turn a 'good' day into a 'bad' day where all bets on eating were off.

At the heart of the Programme are the lifelong changes that free you from a dieter's mindset of 'good' and 'bad' days. In our groups, we explore this idea by talking about John Wooden, one of the greatest US college basketball coaches, celebrated for his powerful wisdom, which spoke to his players' outlook and attitude.

'Make each day your masterpiece' is one of Coach Wooden's most famous sayings.

I like to think that Coach meant, whatever you are doing today, give it your all and do it to the best of your ability. If your eating doesn't go completely to plan, rather than writing off the day as a 'bad day', you can instead see this as a brushstroke on your masterpiece that didn't quite work out. Rather than abandoning your painting, you can decide to keep going, just as a 'naturally' lean person would. The day remains a good day. Today can *still* be your masterpiece.

Secret 7: Sometimes being 'naturally' lean results from feeling good inside

When my patients lose weight and are living the life of a 'naturally' lean person, they find that it is not their weight loss that makes them happy; in fact it's the reverse. It is their new-found healthier inner life, in which they value and care for themselves, that makes them happy and their weight loss is a natural result of this.

Similarly, my happiest patients are often my most successful. Rather than waiting until they reach their final weight target, they are instead living life to the full along the way. Like Mark, whose words open this chapter. Mark hasn't yet reached his goal weight, but this hasn't stopped him from fulfilling his dream of starting a new life in Shetland. By using his Programme tools, Mark understood that life is not a dress rehearsal and that happiness is available to him today, *while* he is on his journey. Mark's approach is also *yours* for the taking. When you use your Programme choices to look after yourself in the here-and-now, you too will develop a new inner-contentment from which even more weight loss will naturally flow.

Secret 8: 'Naturally' lean people write their own stories

We all live our lives according to certain scripts – as Shakespeare pointed out: 'All the world's a stage . . .' We might be living by a 'caregiver' script. Or we might have been handed the script of the 'responsible' eldest in the family or the 'funny' friend. Very often we are playing multiple parts, but in some cases these parts might not suit the life we want to lead.

Through their Programme successes, my patients have taught me that we can be the author of our own story. In your own journey towards becoming a 'naturally' lean person, like my patients, you too can discard any scripts that are holding you back and instead choose new scripts that set you up for a full life.

The story of Thomas Edison gives us a good example of rewriting the script. As a boy, Edison heard a teacher criticizing him, calling him 'addled' – meaning confused, unable to think clearly – and questioning the point of Thomas remaining at the school. When he told his mother, Nancy Edison rejected this script for her son. Rather than allowing him to take on the part of an 'addled' failure, she told the teacher that her son had 'more brains' than *him*. Then she took Edison out of the school and taught him at home herself. You will know that Thomas Edison grew up to be a celebrated and prolific inventor, most famous for his work on the electric light bulb. Mrs Edison rewrote her son's script, creating the part of a boy who was smarter than even his own teacher. 'My mother was the making of me,' Thomas Edison later said.

You don't need a Mrs Edison in your life to rewrite the script. You can do this for yourself. As we do in our groups, if you feel you are playing a part that is not right for you, the next step is to write down this role. You can then read the script for the last time, before tearing up the piece of paper. Next, take a fresh piece of paper and start to write a new script. Write down the part that *you* have chosen to play. Just as my patients have done, you can embrace that new script, begin to learn your lines and choose to play that new part every day.

As you start to enjoy all the benefits of your Programme choices, you might find that playing the part of a 'lucky' person is a natural choice. This will become self-fulfilling because lucky people make their own luck. Their wide focus allows them to notice new opportunities, like using all the tools in this book, which lead to even more lucky outcomes. As you feel good and lose weight, you'll develop the optimism typical of lucky people – a lens through which they view the future as a bright place that's full of possibilities.

When he was choosing his generals, it is said that Napoleon would ask, 'Is he lucky . . . ? Bring me lucky generals.' Napoleon knew what he was talking about. Lucky generals win wars just as lucky Programme participants achieve the things that they want. By embracing all their new choices, they enjoy an inner ease and a belief that good things usually happen to them in a life being lived to the full.

Epilogue:
Look up at the stars . . .

Once my patients have completed their fourteen Programme sessions, we get together one last time to celebrate how far they have come and all that they have achieved. As it says on the medals that they receive in that final graduation session, they have become Programme Champions.

Mixed in with their richly deserved pride, some of my patients feel a sense of sadness that the Programme has come to an end. In fact, as we remind each other, nothing has ended. Their Programme graduation, like you finishing this book, is just the beginning.

I wish I could hold a final celebratory session for you, but instead I can leave you with your complete **Programme Toolkit**. I hope that you will use it to create a future full of good health, living life at the weight that you want to be.

1. **Insulin is the fat controller**. You can keep insulin levels low by eating real, unprocessed foods that do not quickly break down into sugar. Food that your body (and your grandma) would recognize as food.
2. You can tune in to your body's **hunger–fullness messages**, allowing you to eat when you are hungry and stop when you are full.

3. An **Eating Window** allows you to harness the powerful health advantages of choosing *when* you eat.

4. **Feeding your gut bacteria** with foods that are high in fibre, fermented and a rainbow of different colours will support their work to **keep you lean**.

5. Regular daily **movement will melt away insulin resistance**, you will lose weight and improve your health. Your mood will feel brighter too.

6. **Sleeping well** will help you lose weight and improve your physical and mental health.

7. You might have **weight-gain genes**, which are simply the loaded gun. You can choose **not to pull the trigger** by avoiding ultra-processed, sugary foods.

8. **Your health is too precious to trust the food industry to look after it.** You can take back control by knowing your ingredients and cooking your own food. No chemicals, no tricks – just food.

9. You can **use the lessons of history** to recognize that weight gain and illnesses like diabetes are not 'just one of those things'. Rather, through your Programme lifestyle changes you are tackling the root cause of these issues. You have the ownership.

10. By using the **language of success** you can leverage your brain's biology to build new behaviours that make your health and weight-loss goals possible.

11. You are more likely to achieve your **goals** if you know exactly *what* you want, and *where*, *when* and

how you will make it happen. You can search 'MyProgrammeGoals.com', 'place your order', then track its progress and use the power of visualization to see your order 'fulfilled and delivered'.

12. If there could be **a gain or benefit in staying at a certain weight**, you can ask whether you want to **create new behaviours and different outcomes**.

13. If there are times that you eat when you're not hungry, you can **cut out dopamine-rush foods and use the Programme as a stress-reduction technique** while 'filling up' with your favourite people and situations.

14. You can use the **eight secrets of 'naturally' lean people**:
    1. Eat when you are hungry; stop when you are full.
    2. Eat slowly.
    3. 'Sit with' your hunger for a short time if Programme food isn't immediately available.
    4. Use NEAT to keep moving.
    5. Avoid learning from unhealthy TOFI lean people.
    6. Free yourself from a dieter's catastrophizing mindset – today is *still* your masterpiece.
    7. Use your Programme tools to care for and value yourself, and your weight loss will naturally follow.
    8. Write your own story. Live the life you want to lead according to your own script.

I am confident you will be able to successfully use the powerful Butterfly Effect of these fourteen Programme tools. A change in one area (turning your back on ultra-processed food – the butterfly flapping its wings) can produce a big effect on something that is seemingly unrelated (your sleep improving – a tornado far across the world).

I won't tell you that the route to weight loss is always easy. Like my patients, you might hit bumps in the road along the way. I think this is true of anything that you want to achieve in life. When we reach a crossroads we can either choose to be like the other runners or we can, like Roger Bannister, believe that the destination that we seek is still possible.

In the final part of our Programme graduation, when we discuss how to deal with these challenges, we look to the wisdom of one of the great scientists of the modern age – Professor Stephen Hawking.

At 21, Hawking was diagnosed with a degenerative neurological condition. His mobility deteriorated and he soon became wheelchair bound. When he lost the ability to speak he used a computer to synthesize his voice. He never allowed his illness to stop him ceaselessly pushing forward our knowledge of the universe, making a stunning success of his life in which he was celebrated for his game-changing work on the physics of black holes.

In 2012, to a packed Cambridge University lecture theatre, in a speech to mark his seventieth birthday (a milestone many thought he would not live to see), Professor Hawking shared this advice:

**'Remember to look up at the stars and not down
at your feet. Try to make sense of what you see
and wonder about what makes the universe
exist. Be curious. And however difficult life may
seem, there is always something you can do and
succeed at. It matters that you don't just give up.'**

I often think of these words, particularly when facing a challenge. In 2020, when I was redeployed to my hospital's Covid-19 frontline, walking out of a shift I would physically tilt my head back to look up at the vast expanse of night sky above. It felt better than looking down at my feet.

As my patients before you have found, the road ahead will be paved with uncertainty and setbacks, but also with hope, change and soaring successes. This is life in all its technicolour messiness. As you chart your own course, perhaps return to Professor Hawking's words as a final Programme tool – a talisman for the bright and full future ahead of you:

**'Look up at the stars and not down at your feet
. . . it matters that you don't just give up.'**

Full steam ahead:
even more know-how
for your Programme journey

Programme FAQs

Through many years of running the Programme, I have been asked hundreds of questions by my patients. I have compiled the most frequently asked questions and I hope that these answers are valuable to you too.

1. Q: How rigidly should I be sticking to the food lists? Is there any room for manoeuvre here?

A: How you interpret the guidance is very much your choice. Many of my patients have found following the lists works well for them because they are enjoying delicious, filling food, are in control of their eating and, at the same time, are losing weight and feeling good. For example, they are no longer bloated, their acid reflux disappears, their sleep improves and their mood is brighter. So initially, I would advise following the lists as written to reap all of these benefits.

In the future, depending on individual considerations, like how much weight you want to lose, you might want to trial reintroducing certain other foods (see pages 23–4 in Chapter 1 and pages 117–9 in Chapter 7). These foods would still fulfil our criteria of being unprocessed and made with natural ingredients. You can then judge whether tailoring the Programme works for you. You could find that reintroducing some foods is fine but others make you bloated, give you an energy slump or stall your weight loss. As always with the Programme, it's about listening to what your body is telling you.

2. Q: I understand the idea of choosing food that my grandparents would recognize as food, but my grandma ate potatoes, so how does that fit in with the guidance?
A: When making food choices, yes, we like foods that are unprocessed and straightforward. But the second consideration is whether a food will be broken down by the body into a large amount of sugar. So although potatoes are a natural, single-ingredient food, if you eat an average-sized portion of boiled potatoes (about 150g), the effect on your blood sugar levels will be the equivalent of 9 teaspoons of sugar. You will then produce insulin and some of that sugar will be swept into fat, resulting in weight gain. So the unpronounceable, dubious ingredient principle is a helpful guide, but please use this alongside the Choose to Eat List (see pages 20–2) and the Choose Not to Eat List (see pages 24–5).

The second part of my answer relates to how our grandparents ate unprocessed foods like potatoes and remained at a healthy weight. The background here is that the extent to which high-carbohydrate foods, like potatoes, rice, bread and pasta, lead to weight gain will depend on how active you are and your degree of insulin resistance.

Given the era she was living in, your grandma probably wasn't insulin resistant because she ate in a certain way and was physically active. When she ate potatoes, she will have needed less insulin to sweep the excess sugar out of the blood because her body was responsive to insulin (there was no resistance to overcome). Her healthy insulin response meant that potatoes were less pro-fat storing in her than they would be in those of us with insulin resistance.

This dovetails with the first question about reintroducing certain foods in the future. As your insulin resistance falls through your Programme changes, you will produce less insulin in response to these foods, making them less pro-weight gain than they were when you were insulin resistant.

3. Q: Are these ingredients/is this food OK?

A: This question summarizes the many questions I am asked by my patients about specific foods and ingredients. I have summarized the answers that I have given over the years as the following two-step guide:

i. The very best Programme foods have no ingredients. For example, eggs are eggs and apples are apples. No labels, no decoding required.
ii. The Programme does include pre-prepared foods, like mayonnaise, pesto and hummus. Importantly, these are all foods that it's possible for us to make at home, which means the food is less likely to have been subjected to ultra-processing techniques. Here, checking the ingredients list is key. Please make sure

the ingredients sound like food. If we take pesto as an example, this should contain olive oil, basil, Parmesan cheese, cashew or pine nuts, garlic and salt. When you are checking an ingredients list, the food is likely to be fine if, as in this example, it contains recognizable, pronounceable ingredients that a home cook would use.

4. Q: I like to have an afternoon snack. Please can you recommend snacks that would work well with the Programme?
A: Here are some suggestions for delicious Programme snacks:
• Cherry tomatoes with cheese
• Chopped crudités, such as cucumber, carrots and celery with a dip like hummus or tzatziki
• One or two boiled eggs
• Sliced cold cuts, such as chicken, turkey or ham with full-fat cream cheese
• Olives
• Turkey or ham roll-ups (see Super-speedy recipes on page 286)
• Nuts (not salted or processed) – a handful
• An apple with a couple of teaspoons of a nut butter
• Greek yogurt/full-fat natural yogurt – 100 to 200g
• Homemade leftovers

5. Q: We're going away at the weekend – please can I ask for some pointers for when I'm away from home?

A: This question covers a variety of situations, from travelling to eating out to visiting someone's home. Here are my top tips for staying on track when you are away from home:

i. If you're planning to be out for much of the day, take food that travels well with you. This will keep you firmly in control of what you are eating. Suggestions include:
   - Veg, like carrots, celery, peppers and cherry tomatoes
   - Fruit, such as berries, apples or pears
   - Nuts
   - Olives
   - Cheese
   - Pre-cooked sausages
   - Boiled eggs
   - Turkey, ham, salami or cold cuts
   - Homemade leftovers

ii. When you go out to a restaurant, unlike with restrictive diets, you'll be eating delicious food – no missing out. Good examples to look for on the menu are fish or meat with vegetables, salads and cheese. Also have a look in the Recipes section (see pages 219–89) as this will give you an idea of the sort of Programme-perfect foods you'll see on restaurant menus.

   Almost every restaurant will make changes when you ask. For example, if there's steak and chips on the menu, you can ask to swap the chips for a salad, buttered greens or roasted vegetables. You might worry about speaking up and asking for substitutions – some of my patients initially felt that way too. However, they found

that restaurants and hotels were happy to help so they
enjoyed a great meal that fuelled their body correctly.

iii. If you are having coffee or afternoon tea at someone's
house, bring something as a gift like a fruit platter or the
chocolate truffles from the Recipes section (page 279).

iv. When you are invited to someone's house for lunch or
dinner, tell them in advance about how you are choosing
to eat. Remember, people want you to enjoy being at
their home. Once you've told them, your host will be
accommodating, just as they would be if you said you
were vegetarian or had other reasons for being specific
about your food choices.

**6. Q: I have cleared out my kitchen as you suggested
but have kept organic coconut sugar, is this a good
idea?**

A: Sugar is sugar and organic coconut sugar is just sugar
with better branding. The same applies to brown sugar,
jaggery and liquid sugars, like agave syrup/nectar, honey
(including Manuka honey) and maple syrup. All of these
will spike your blood sugar levels just like ordinary,
standard cane sugar, and some of the sugar will end up
in fat stores.

You've also raised a very good point here with regards
to organic foods. Many people are under the impression
that if something is organic then it must be healthy. In fact,
organic simply describes the farming methods rather than
the health qualities of the food.

7. Q: I often make fruit and veg smoothies and juices. How does this fit into the Programme?

A: Smoothies and juices are sugar solutions. Through the juicing process, water and sugar (the juice/smoothie) are extracted, while the fibre is broken up by the blending (and, in the case of juice, usually thrown away in the pulp). The difference between eating an apple and drinking apple juice makes this point. A whole apple contains 3g of fibre and when you eat an apple as a fruit, the equivalent of 2 teaspoons of sugar will end up in your blood. Compare this to a 200ml glass of apple juice in which most of the fibre has been removed by the juicing, so the juice contains only a third of the fibre of the whole apple (1g). When you drink the juice, the equivalent of 9 teaspoons of sugar will end up in your blood. Not only is this a low-fibre meal for your gut bacteria, the sugar in juice and smoothies will also put you into fat-storage mode.

8. Q: Can I do the Programme if I am vegetarian?

A: Yes! I have had many vegetarian patients who have enjoyed lots of Programme success. As you can see from the Choose to Eat List (pages 20–2), sample menu (page 290) and recipe ideas (pages 219–89), there are many options for you if you are vegetarian. These choices also speak to those of us who aren't vegetarian but are looking to eat more plant-based foods.

9. Q: Are non-dairy milk alternatives, like nut milks, a good choice if they don't contain odd ingredients?

A: Some non-dairy alternatives to milk have dubious ingredients, while others are straightforward. For example, there are some good almond milks that just contain almonds, water and sea salt. All pronounceable, all recognizable – fine to add to your Programme food choices.

10. Q: What do you think of gluten-free bread?
A: Gluten free simply means that the food does not contain the protein gluten. The effect of the bread being broken down by the body into sugar is still the same, so it is not a recommended food for our low-sugar way of eating. What's more, without gluten, all sorts of fillers and thickeners are often added to mimic the texture and structure that gluten gives to bread. These ingredients mean we have to be vigilant with products labelled gluten-free – the ingredients list can be pretty alarming.

11. Q: Are raisins, dates and other dried fruits part of the Programme?
A: Gram for gram, raisins, dates and other dried fruits contain as much sugar as a chocolate bar. Dried fruits will therefore result in high insulin levels, which will lead to fat storage and weight gain.

12. Q: Why are certain fruits preferred over others?
Fruits like berries are suggested because they are low sugar, which means low levels of insulin and less sweeping into fat storage.

The word dessert originally referred to the fruit course

at grand dinners, which is a helpful reminder for how sweet fruit is. At the time, most people ate relatively little sugar, so fruit, when it was available, tasted very sweet. I use this 'dessert' context as a reminder that some fruits, like bananas, grapes, mangoes and pineapple, are especially high in sugar. On the other hand, the fruits we choose on the Programme are low or medium sugar and will keep your blood sugar levels stable and your insulin levels controlled.

13. Q: I'm curious about the reference to portion size in the food list. I realize we are not counting calories but do we acknowledge portion limits?

A: Having been on and off diets for years, many of my patients join the Programme unsure about what hunger and fullness means any more. Advising on portions and servings (see the Choose to Eat List on pages 20–2 and the Recipes section on pages 219–89) helps with this recalibration. Later on, when people get up and running, they can eat when they're hungry and stop when they're full, but initially these benchmarks will help to get them there.

Some people who have been eating a carbohydrate-heavy diet are used to the stomach stretch of these starchy foods as a guide to when to stop eating. Programme foods do not produce that uneasy stuffed feeling, so some of my patients take a bit of time to find other cues that they've eaten enough. Having some guidance on portions and amounts helps with this.

Lastly, the Programme recommends choosing to eat food like cheese, nuts and full-fat milk that many people will have avoided for years. So it's important initially to get your eye in with what a regular amount of these foods looks like. All foods – whether carbohydrate or not – result in a rise in blood sugar. A piece of cheese will result in a far smaller rise in blood sugar than a piece of toast but eating a lot of cheese in one go will require insulin to deal with it; and unless you keep your insulin levels low, you can't break down your fat stores and lose weight. The Programme is a low-sugar–low-insulin plan, not an unlimited eating plan. When you are getting up and running with your food choices, portion guides help to establish this.

14. Q: You recommended closing the Eating Window for about sixteen hours. Can I close it for longer than this?
A: As ever, this comes down to what feels right for you. The evidence suggests that you will achieve the benefits of the Eating Window by closing for sixteen hours. However, if the ebb and flow of your own ghrelin hunger signal and your daily routine means that closing for longer than sixteen hours suits you, then of course you can choose to do this.

15. Q: Is there a best time of day to exercise?
A: All exercise, any time, is good, the one caveat being exercise close to bedtime, which releases stimulatory hormones like adrenaline that can interfere with falling asleep.
   If you exercise first thing, while your Eating Window is still closed, by this time in the morning your body will have

used up the fuel stores in your liver and muscles so will tap into the energy in your fat stores to power your exercise.

Alternatively, if you choose to exercise when your Eating Window is open, this will bring down your blood sugar levels because the sugar in your blood from the food you have eaten will be used immediately by your muscles, lungs and heart instead of being stored in fat for future use.

16. Q: Should I load up on certain foods before exercise? And when I finish, is it better to have a protein shake or a sports drink?

A: Whether you need to eat before exercise depends on what you're doing. For most exercise, like going for a walk or cycling as part of your commute, then the answer is no – your body's fuel stores will give you all the energy that you need. If you are going to be exercising for a long time, like a triathlon or a long run, then you might choose to eat something in advance.

The second part of your question taps into the commonly held view of the need to 'replenish' or 'recover' after exercise with sports drinks, bars, gels or protein shakes. If you have been using these products, please take a look at the ingredients list, which is likely to be full of sugar or artificial sweeteners, flavourings and other dubious ingredients. Even if you find a product that is fairly straightforward, it isn't *food* as we understand it in the Programme. If you feel the need to eat after exercise, then I would advise choosing to eat *food* over these ultra-processed sports-branded products.

17. Q: How much weight should I expect to lose and how quickly will I see results?

A: On average, our patients lose 14 per cent of their body weight. Some lose less than this and some significantly more. Some have lost 25 per cent of their body weight, which is similar to the weight loss seen after gastric bypass surgery.

You can use this calculation to work out what a 14 per cent weight loss looks like:

0.14 (which is 14 per cent) × your current weight

Let's say you are 14 stone 2lb (90kg) now. Your numbers would be:

0.14 × 90 = 12.6kg (which is 27.8lb – approximately a 2-stone weight loss)

These weight-loss percentages have to be taken in context and in particular your own weight loss will depend on your starting weight and how much weight you are looking to lose. If you start the Programme at 11 stone (70kg) wanting to lose a stone (6.4kg), this will be 9 per cent of your body weight – which will be the weight-loss success that you want.

The rate of weight loss is very variable between people and can be anything from 1lb to sometimes as much as 6lb (0.5kg to 3kg) a week. You should see results within the first week of starting the Programme, which gives a real momentum boost to keep on going.

18. Q: My weight loss has stalled for the last three weeks, what can I do about this?

A: The first thing to ask yourself is, 'What was I doing before?' This means reviewing all of your fourteen tools (there's a useful summary on pages 194–6) as well as the choices at the end of the chapters. This will allow you to reflect on whether you are still doing the things you were doing when your weight was falling. For example, are you still keeping to your Eating Window timings and are you moving every day? It's also a good idea to check if you are still following the Choose to Eat List (pages 20–2) and also to consider whether your portion sizes have changed. I don't usually like food diaries because we all live in the real world and they can be inconvenient to keep. This is the only instance, though, when I suggest that my patients make a note on their phone for three days of what they are eating (including the amount) and when (the times) they are eating. You can also record your daily movement and how much sleep you are getting. When it comes to a weight-loss stall (or even a regain) this diary can be illuminating for identifying if anything has gone off-track and how to fix it.

If your weight plateaus for a period of time, it's also important to bear in mind that the Programme weight-loss pattern is not a straight downward slope. Rather, there will be some weeks when you lose and some weeks where you stay the same. Here, please remember that maintaining is also a win. Sometimes my patients feel discouraged if their weight remains the same from one week to the next. If this happens, I ask them to reflect on all the non-weight related benefits they are achieving, like having more energy, a brighter mood and being fully in control of their eating. The number falling on the scales of course feels great, but it is just one part of many other feel-good Programme outcomes.

Shopping list ideas

This is not a list to buy all at once! Rather, it is a guide to choose from depending on your eating plans. My patients have found it very helpful for navigating their food shopping, particularly when they are first getting started in the Programme. These shopping list ideas also help to create, over time, a go-to store cupboard and freezer of handy ingredients that can be used again and again in your delicious Programme cooking.

FRESH VEGETABLES AND FRUIT
- Fresh vegetables – for example, baby corn, broccoli, Brussels sprouts, cabbage, cauliflower, celeriac, green beans, kale, mushrooms, runner beans and spinach
- Green salad leaves, such as lettuce, pak choi, rocket and Chinese leaf
- Stir-fry vegetable mix
- Carrots, celery, cucumber and radishes
- Aubergines, courgettes, peppers (any colour) and tomatoes
- Avocados
- Onions, shallots, leeks and garlic
- Fruit, such as blueberries, raspberries, strawberries, apples, pears, lemons and limes

EGGS

DAIRY
- Whole, full-fat milk

- Full-fat natural (plain) or Greek yogurt
- Kefir (check it only has two ingredients – milk and beneficial bacteria cultures)
- Cheese, such as Cheddar, feta, halloumi, mozzarella, Parmesan and cream cheese
- Cream – single, double or clotted
- Full-fat crème fraîche
- Butter – salted or unsalted, depending on your preference
- Non-dairy milk alternatives (check the ingredients are straightforward and non-dubious – for example, an almond milk should contain almonds, water and sometimes sea salt)

MEAT

- Any kind of fresh meat – for example, chicken legs or thighs (skin on), whole chicken for roasting, turkey, beef mince, beef steak, lamb, pork (check there's no breading, sauces or dubious ingredients, just one ingredient – meat!)
- Bacon
- Sausages – pork, beef, chicken or lamb with a high meat content, which means more than 90 per cent meat
- Sliced ham or turkey (with no added sugar, honey, syrups or breading)
- Antipasto selection – for example, prosciutto and salami
- Pâté (with no added sugar, only containing pronounceable ingredients)

FISH

- Any fresh fish and shellfish (no breading, no sauces, just one ingredient – fish!)
- Smoked salmon – slices or trimmings

GENERAL

- Hummus
- Tzatziki

- Guacamole
- Fresh olives
- Tofu

STORE CUPBOARD:

- Olive oil
- Salt and pepper
- Dried herbs and spices – for example, chilli powder, chipotle, oregano, dried mint, sumac, piri piri, jerk, ras el hanout (for the mixtures, check they contain no added sugar)
- Raw unsalted nuts – for example, Brazil nuts, pecans, walnuts, almonds, macadamias and pistachios
- Nut butters, such as peanut butter, almond butter and hazelnut butter (check there is no added sugar and they are palm-oil free)
- Seeds – for example, flaxseed (also known as linseed), pumpkin seeds, sesame seeds, sunflower seeds and hemp seeds
- Passata
- Tomato purée
- Tinned tomatoes – chopped or whole
- Tinned tuna
- Jar of pesto
- Jar of sundried tomatoes
- Artichokes in olive oil
- Peppers in olive oil
- Olives – tinned or in a jar
- Soy sauce (check that there are no odd ingredients – something along the lines of soya beans, water and salt is ideal)
- Vinegar, such as white wine vinegar or apple cider vinegar
- Tahini (sesame seed paste)
- Sauerkraut

- Arrowroot powder
- Ground linseed or flaxseed
- Lentils – dried or tinned
- Tinned chickpeas
- Tinned sweetcorn (no added sugar – two ingredients: sweetcorn and water)
- Full-fat mayonnaise (check for any dubious ingredients)
- 85% or 90% dark chocolate
- Herbal tea (such as camomile or mint) or fruit tea
- Tea and coffee

FREEZER

- Frozen berries – for example, raspberries, blueberries, strawberries and mixed berries
- Frozen spinach
- Frozen green beans
- Frozen cauliflower florets
- Frozen cauliflower rice
- Frozen broccoli florets
- Frozen peas
- Frozen chopped onions
- Frozen garlic
- Frozen ginger
- Frozen red chilli
- Frozen chicken – legs, thighs or breast – skin on, if possible (no breading or added ingredients, just one ingredient – chicken!)
- Frozen fish – for example, cod, salmon and fish pie mix (no breading or added ingredients, just one ingredient – fish!)
- Frozen prawns

Recipes

These are some of my favourite Programme recipes, cooked and enjoyed by my patients and their families and friends over many years. I am certain they will bring you great pleasure too, as well as nourishment for your body and soul – no chemicals, no hacks, no tricks.

One of my favourite things about the Programme is how it harnesses the power of eating delicious, real food to lose weight and reclaim your health. As you'll see when you try out these recipes, the Programme will reconnect you with the joy of food and eating. These recipes look and taste so good that if you throw a party and serve any of these dishes, your guests will have no idea that you are on any sort of plan and will simply compliment you on how well you eat.

These recipes contain something for everyone. There are vegetarian and vegan options, as well as plenty of scope to be flexible on the ingredients. The recipes have been carefully designed for you to fine-tune so that the tastes and flavours are perfect for you. Some recipes can be prepared in minutes for a quick mid-week meal. Others ask for a bit more time to build up the layers of flavour. But in all cases, the recipes have been designed for real life. They don't require unusual kitchen equipment and only use ingredients that are routinely available yet burst with taste and flavour. I've indicated which recipes make particularly convenient portable foods and which ones can be batch cooked ahead of time. Importantly, I have highlighted options for cutting down on food waste so that we use and enjoy as much of the food as possible.

Some of my patients who joined the Programme uncertain of their cooking skills were bowled over by the dishes that they created; and as their confidence in the kitchen grew, so did their repertoire. Talk in our group was alive with the buzz of shared know-how and new ideas, while at the same time their weight was falling and their happiness was soaring. I am certain that these recipes will bring you the same sense of satisfaction and pleasure. Happy cooking and happy eating!

SCRAMBLED EGGS WITH SMOKED SALMON, MUSHROOMS AND SPINACH

ready in under 15 / vegetarian option

Serves 2
Takes 10 minutes
Hands-on: 5 minutes / Hands-off: 5 minutes

20g butter
200g chestnut mushrooms (or mushroom of choice),
    thinly sliced
120g baby spinach
4 large eggs
3 tablespoons double cream or whole milk
1 tablespoon chives (optional), finely chopped
120g smoked salmon (optional)
salt and black pepper

Heat half the butter in a non-stick frying pan until melted and bubbling. Add the sliced mushrooms and a little seasoning and cook for 3–4 minutes on a high heat, shaking occasionally, until they are lightly golden. Remove from the pan and keep warm.

Reduce the heat to medium and add the spinach and a tablespoon of water. Stir until the spinach has just wilted. This should only take a minute or two, then remove from the pan and add to the mushrooms. As you transfer the spinach, give it a gentle squeeze to make sure any excess water is removed.

Turn the heat right down and add the remaining butter to the pan. Crack the eggs into a jug and beat with the cream or milk and some seasoning. Add to the pan once the butter has started to smell a little nutty. Stir gently until cooked to your liking and then stir in the chives.

Divide the salmon (if using) between two plates, followed by the scrambled eggs, mushrooms and spinach.

TIP

If you are using smoked salmon, the small packets come in different weights – often 100g or 120g – use whichever you can find. Smoked salmon trimmings will also work well.

THE ONE-PAN FULL MONTY

Serves 2
Takes 25 minutes
Hands-on: 15 minutes / Hands-off: 10 minutes

2 tablespoons olive oil
4 rashers of unsmoked back bacon
6 asparagus spears (optional), ends snapped off and
   spears sliced in half lengthways
10 cherry tomatoes, sliced in half
6 chestnut mushrooms (or mushroom of choice), thinly
   sliced
4 slices of halloumi cheese
4 large eggs
a pinch of chilli flakes
salt and black pepper

Take a large frying pan and place on a medium-low heat. Add
1 tablespoon of the oil and when hot, add the bacon on one
side, cooking for around 8 minutes. Turn it occasionally until
the fat has gone golden brown and the bacon is cooked.

On the other half of the pan add the asparagus (if using)
and tomatoes. Season generously and cook until both have
just softened. Remove along with the bacon and keep warm.

Pour the remaining oil into the pan and add the mushrooms on one side and the halloumi on the other. Cook the
halloumi for a couple of minutes on each side until golden

brown and the mushrooms are done to your liking. Remove and keep with the bacon.

There should still be enough oil in the pan, but if need be you can add another teaspoon and crack in the four eggs. Fry to your liking, adding a pinch of chilli flakes to the top of each along with salt and pepper while cooking and then you are ready to serve.

Divide the bacon, asparagus, tomatoes, mushrooms, halloumi and eggs between two plates and eat while hot.

TURKISH BAKED EGGS

vegetarian

Serves 2
Takes 25 minutes
Hands-on: 15 minutes / Hands-off: 10 minutes

2 tablespoons olive oil
1 large red onion, diced
1 red pepper, deseeded and diced
3 cloves of garlic, sliced
1 tablespoon tomato purée
400g tin of plum or chopped tomatoes
2 teaspoons sumac or zest of a lemon
1 teaspoon chilli flakes
2 tablespoons chopped parsley
2 tablespoons chopped coriander
4 large eggs
salt and black pepper

Pour the oil into a large frying pan on a medium heat and add the onion, pepper and garlic. Cook, stirring occasionally, for 10 minutes until everything has softened and started to go golden brown.

Add the tomato purée and stir into the onion mix. Then add the tinned tomatoes and break them up with the spoon (if using plum tomatoes). Turn the heat down and cook for 5–6 minutes until the sauce starts thickening.

Add the sumac or lemon zest, chilli flakes and fresh herbs with some seasoning and mix well.

Make four wells in the mix and crack in the eggs. Pop a lid on the pan and cook for 5 minutes or until the eggs are cooked to your liking.

Add a final twist of black pepper and serve hot from the pan.

TIP

If you buy fresh herbs for this recipe, you can chop any leftovers and freeze in an ice-cube tray with a little oil.

FETA AND RED ONION EGG MUFFINS

vegetarian / great portable option / batch cook

Makes 12 (one serving is 2)
Takes 30 minutes
Hands-on: 10 minutes / Hands-off: 20 minutes

2 tablespoons olive oil
1 large red onion, thinly sliced
2 cloves of garlic, finely grated
100g baby spinach
6 large eggs
75g feta (or mature Cheddar), crumbled
2 tablespoons dried oregano
80ml double cream
salt and black pepper

Preheat the oven to 180°C/160°C fan/gas 4 and use a little butter or olive oil to grease a non-stick 12-hole muffin tin (silicone moulds or cases are excellent for this).

Pour the olive oil into a frying pan, add the red onion and garlic and cook for 8 minutes until softened and starting to go golden brown. Add the spinach and stir into the onion until wilted. You don't want any water to be coming out of the spinach, so cook until there is none.

Remove the pan from the heat and keep to one side while you crack the eggs into a large mixing jug. Beat well with a fork and then add the feta, oregano, double cream, a pinch of salt and a good twist of black pepper. Mix well with a fork and then add the onion mix.

Beat everything together and pour even amounts into each of the muffin tin holes, or silicon cases if using, filling to around a centimetre from the top (or else they spill over).

Place the tin in the hot oven. Bake for 15 minutes until golden, risen and cooked all the way through.

Remove from the oven, allow to cool for 5 minutes and then remove to a wire rack to cool fully if not eating immediately.

Delicious served with a green salad or any other Programme vegetables of your choosing

TIP

> You can make these in advance and reheat. They are also great to have as a lunch-on-the-go as they are just as tasty cold!

BROCCOLI AND BLUE CHEESE SOUP

vegetarian / batch cook

Serves 4
Takes 35 minutes
Hands-on: 15 minutes / Hands-off: 20 minutes

    1 tablespoon olive oil
    10g unsalted butter
    1 large leek, sliced
    3 celery stalks, sliced
    3 cloves of garlic, sliced
    2 bay leaves
    500g broccoli, chopped into florets
    800ml vegetable stock (or bouillon)
    150ml whole milk
    150g creamy blue cheese (like Stilton, Gorgonzola,
       Cambozola) or Cheddar, diced or grated
    salt and black pepper

To serve (optional)
    extra virgin olive oil
    Parmesan shavings

Heat the olive oil and butter in a large saucepan and add the
leek, celery, garlic and bay leaves. Cook for 5–10 minutes
until the leek has softened and the garlic is just starting to go
golden brown.

Add the broccoli and stir to mix. Season with a little salt and pepper and then add the vegetable stock. Bring up to a simmer and cook for 20 minutes or until the broccoli stalks are soft.

Add the milk and cheese and stir until the cheese has melted.

Remove from the heat and either use a stick blender or transfer to a counter-top blender or food processor and blitz until smooth. Check the seasoning and adjust to taste.

Serve with a drizzle of extra virgin olive oil, a last flourish of black pepper and a few Parmesan shavings.

Delicious with an accompaniment of crunchy freshly chopped crudités like carrots and celery.

TIP

This soup is ideal for batch cooking if you double the quantities and will last in the fridge for 3–4 days.

THAI CAULIFLOWER AND COCONUT SOUP

vegan option

Serves 4
Takes 40 minutes
Hands-on: 15 minutes / Hands-off: 25 minutes

1 tablespoon coconut oil
2 banana shallots, chopped
2 cloves of garlic, chopped
3cm piece of ginger, peeled and chopped
1 stick of lemongrass (optional – will really lift the dish if available), end trimmed, outer leaf removed and sliced
700g whole cauliflower (approx. 1 large), roughly chopped into 2cm pieces
1 tablespoon fish sauce (vegan option available if preferred)
1–2 teaspoons chilli flakes
400ml tin of coconut milk (look for a high percentage of coconut solids with no additives)
zest and juice of a lime
1 tablespoon chopped coriander

Heat the coconut oil in a large saucepan and then add the shallot, garlic, ginger and lemongrass and cook for 5 minutes. At this point everything should be really aromatic and that's the sign to add the cauliflower.

Stir to mix everything together and then add the fish sauce, chilli flakes, coconut milk and 400ml cold water. Bring up to a simmer and then reduce the heat. Cook for 20–25 minutes until the cauliflower core is very soft.

Remove from the heat and use a stick blender or transfer to a counter-top blender or food processor and blitz until smooth.

Once you are happy with the consistency, add the lime zest, lime juice and coriander. Stir through and serve.

TIP

You can freeze leftover lemongrass sticks for future use.

GREEK SALAD

ready in under 15 / vegetarian

Serves 2 as a main meal or 4 as a side dish
Takes 10 minutes

½ cucumber, cut into chunks
2 large tomatoes, cut into chunks
1 green pepper, deseeded and cut into chunks
1 small red onion, diced
2 tablespoons chopped parsley
2 tablespoons dried oregano
1 teaspoon sumac or zest of a lemon
200g feta, crumbled
10 black pitted olives (fresh or tinned/jarred), cut in half
juice of a lemon
3 tablespoons extra virgin olive oil
salt and black pepper

Place the cucumber, tomato, pepper, onion, parsley, oregano
and sumac (or lemon zest) into a bowl and toss gently to
combine.

Crumble in the feta and add the olives.

Drizzle over the lemon juice, extra virgin olive oil and
season to taste with salt and pepper. Give it another good
mix before serving.

CHICKEN TIKKA SALAD

Serves 2

Takes 25 minutes

Hands-on: 15 minutes / Hands-off: 10 minutes

For the chicken
>   2 large chicken thighs (boneless, skin on or off depending
>   on preference)
>   60g full-fat Greek yogurt
>   juice of ½ lemon
>   1 heaped teaspoon tikka masala paste (with no added
>   sugar or preservatives)

For the salad
>   1 romaine lettuce, shredded
>   ½ cucumber, thinly sliced with a peeler
>   10 cherry tomatoes, halved
>   1 avocado, sliced

For the dressing
>   juice of ½ lemon
>   2 tablespoons extra virgin olive oil
>   1 teaspoon dried mint
>   salt and black pepper

Preheat your grill to its highest setting and let it get really
hot.

Place the chicken thighs in a mixing bowl and add the Greek yogurt, lemon juice and tikka masala paste. Stir to mix and coat the chicken.

Line a shallow baking sheet with tin foil and place the chicken on it. Place under the hot grill for 8 minutes each side. You should be starting to get some really good colour on the bits closest to the grill by this point. Add another couple of minutes if needed.

While the chicken is cooking, put the lettuce, cucumber and tomatoes into a bowl and toss to combine. Transfer to a serving plate and then add the avocado slices.

Whisk together in a small bowl the remaining lemon juice, extra virgin olive oil, dried mint and seasoning. Drizzle over the salad.

Remove the hot chicken from the grill, slice and place on top of the salad.

TUNA NIÇOISE SALAD

ready in under 15

Serves 2
Takes 15 minutes
Hands-on: 10 minutes / Hands-off: 5 minutes

For the salad
    3 large eggs
    100g green beans
    1 romaine lettuce (or lettuce of choice), shredded
    1 red onion, thinly sliced (optional)
    12 cherry tomatoes, halved
    2 celery stalks, sliced
    12 black pitted olives (fresh or tinned/jarred), cut in half
    2 × 145g tins of tuna in olive oil

For the dressing
    2 tablespoons olive oil
    1 teaspoon Dijon or wholegrain mustard
    lemon juice, freshly squeezed or bottled (if bottled,
        check it is one ingredient only: lemon juice!)
    salt and black pepper

Bring two pans of water to the boil. Place the eggs in one and cook for 6 minutes for a semi-runny yolk, or 10 minutes if you like it set. Place the green beans in the other pan and cook for 5 minutes until al dente. Once both the eggs and the beans are done, drain and rinse under cold water, then set to one side.

Divide the lettuce between two plates and top each with half the red onion (if using), tomatoes, celery and olives. Peel the eggs and cut in half, giving three halves to each plate. Open the tins of tuna, drain the excess oil and flake over.

Use a small, clean jam jar to shake together the oil, mustard, as much lemon juice as you like (add incrementally) and some seasoning. Drizzle over the salad and enjoy.

TIPS

Alternatively, you can mix the tuna with 2 tablespoons of full-fat mayonnaise and some seasoning to make a tuna mayo, then add to the salad instead of the dressing.

If you save the lemon halves after juicing they can be used in a delicious 'lemonade' – place in a large jug, add sparkling water and leave in the fridge for a few hours to infuse.

ASPARAGUS AND PECORINO ALMOND-BASE TART

vegetarian

Serves 6
Takes 50 minutes
Hands-on: 15 minutes / Hands-off: 30–35 minutes

For the tart base
    250g ground almonds
    75g unsalted butter, at room temperature
    a pinch of salt

For the filling
    100g ricotta cheese
    2 large eggs
    2 egg yolks
    200ml double cream
    100g pecorino cheese (or Parmesan), finely grated
    2 tablespoons chopped tarragon leaves (or 1 tablespoon
        dried tarragon)
    black pepper
    150g asparagus spears, ends snapped off

Preheat the oven to 180°C/160°C fan/gas 4 and line a 20cm loose-bottomed shallow, round tin with baking paper.

    Place the ground almonds, butter and pinch of salt into a mixing bowl and use your hands to rub the butter in, pressing and squeezing until you have a dough.

Shape into a flat round disc with your hands and then lay it in the base of the tin. Gently start to press it out to fill the base and work it up the sides, keeping it as even as possible.

Prick the base with a fork and bake for 15 minutes until golden brown.

While the base is baking, whisk together in a mixing bowl or large jug the ricotta and whole eggs. Once the ricotta is incorporated nicely, add the egg yolks and double cream. Finally, stir in the pecorino, tarragon and a good twist of black pepper. You don't need to add salt as the pecorino is salty enough all by itself.

Pour the egg and cheese mix into the baked almond case and then gently lay the asparagus on top. Bake in the oven for 30–35 minutes until it just has a slight wobble left in the middle.

Remove from the oven and allow to cool for a few minutes before removing from the tin.

Delicious warm, served with green beans or cold with a side salad.

TIP

You can freeze leftover egg whites to use for an egg white omelette or frittata.

FRITTATAS

vegetarian options / great portable option

Serves 6
Takes 30 minutes
Hands-on: 15 minutes / Hands-off: 15 minutes

Option 1: Mushroom, Cheddar and prosciutto
  75g unsalted butter
  1 large red onion, thinly sliced
  300g chestnut mushrooms (or mushroom of choice),
    thinly sliced
  200g baby spinach
  10 large eggs
  200g medium Cheddar, grated
  6 slices of prosciutto (optional)
  salt and black pepper

Option 2: Pea, mint and cheese
  75g unsalted butter
  1 large leek, sliced in half lengthways and cut into 5mm
    half-moons
  200g frozen peas
  1 tablespoon chopped mint
  10 large eggs
  200g goat's cheese (or feta), cut into chunks
  salt and black pepper

Option 3: Red pepper, chorizo and manchego
  75g unsalted butter
  2 red onions, thinly sliced
  2 red peppers, deseeded and cut into chunks
  100g chorizo (optional), diced
  10 large eggs
  1 tablespoon smoked paprika
  1 teaspoon garlic granules
  2 tablespoons chopped parsley
  200g manchego (or Cheddar if you prefer), grated
  salt and black pepper

Preheat the oven to 190°C/170°C fan/gas 5.

For option 1, melt the butter in a deep non-stick, 25cm, oven-compatable frying pan over a medium heat. When it starts to smell nutty, add the onion. Cook for a few minutes until it starts to soften and then add the mushrooms.

Cook on a high heat, stirring often, until the mushrooms stop releasing water and go golden. This will likely take 8–10 minutes. Add the spinach and stir for another minute or two. It should wilt very quickly.

Turn the heat right down, crack the eggs into a large measuring jug and beat well with a fork. Add a good pinch of salt and lots of black pepper and beat to combine.

Add the eggs to the pan along with the Cheddar and gently stir. The egg should slowly start to thicken and resemble the beginnings of scrambled egg. Make sure you are moving all the egg off the base and sides of the pan so it doesn't set too soon.

When it is roughly half cooked, scrunch up the slices of prosciutto and press into the top of the egg. Turn off the heat and pop the pan into the oven for 10–12 minutes to finish cooking.

For option 2, sweat the leek in the butter for 5–8 minutes until softened and then add in the peas for another 2 minutes. Add the mint and beaten egg and when you get to the half-cooked stage, instead of adding prosciutto, add chunks of goat's cheese.

For option 3, sweat the red onion and peppers in the butter for 10 minutes until softened and just starting to go golden. Add in the chorizo (if using) and cook for another 5 minutes. Beat the eggs, adding the paprika, garlic and parsley as you beat. Finally, add the manchego along with the eggs to the pan when the veg is cooked (as you would have added the Cheddar in option 1).

The frittatas are delicious served with a simple green salad or a side of steamed green vegetables.

TIPS

As with all frittatas, the main thing here is to cook your vegetables before you add the eggs. You can leave them slightly underdone so they finish cooking in the egg mix.

If you buy a bunch of mint, you can use any that's left over to make a pot of fresh mint tea. Alternatively, freeze any unused mint as whole leaves in a freezer bag to use another day.

Frittatas are a great way of using up leftover vegetables.

Frittatas are also delicious eaten cold and are a great portable option for a packed lunch or picnic.

SIMPLE DAAL WITH A QUICK PICKLE

batch cook / vegetarian / vegan option

Serves 4
Takes 40 minutes
Hands-on: 15 minutes / Hands-off: 20–25 minutes

For the daal
   300g dried red lentils
   1 tablespoon ghee (or 1 tablespoon olive oil for a vegan
      option)
   8 blocks of frozen spinach
   3 cloves of garlic, grated
   3cm piece of ginger, peeled and grated
   2 teaspoons garam masala
   1 teaspoon chilli flakes (optional)

For the pickle
   1 red onion, diced
   2 tomatoes, deseeded and diced
   ½ cucumber, diced
   1 teaspoon chopped mint leaves
   juice of 1 lemon
   salt and black pepper

To serve
   full-fat natural yogurt

Rinse the lentils in a colander under running water until the water runs clear, then put into a large saucepan. Add one litre of cold water and bring up to the boil. Skim off any scum and then cook at a boil for 10 minutes.

While the lentils are cooking, heat the ghee (or olive oil) in another saucepan. Add the frozen spinach, garlic, ginger, garam masala and chilli flakes (if using) and cook altogether, stirring frequently to help the spinach defrost.

Once the lentils have had 10 minutes, turn the heat down and cook for another 10–15 minutes until very soft and most of the water has been absorbed.

Take the spinach off the heat and stir into the lentils. Continue to cook until it reaches your preferred consistency.

To make the pickle, mix the onion, tomato, cucumber and mint in a bowl and add the lemon juice with a pinch of salt and pepper.

Serve the daal with the pickle and a swirl of natural yogurt.

TIP

You can double the pickle recipe and save half for another time as it makes a delicious accompaniment to many other dishes, including salads, stir-fries or on the side of a mezze platter. The pickle should be stored in the fridge and will last up to 8 weeks.

MEZZE PLATTER

vegetarian options

Serves 2 as a main meal or 4 as a starter
Takes 20 minutes

Butter bean hummus
  400g tin of butter beans, drained and rinsed
  2 tablespoons tahini
  2 tablespoons olive oil
  ½ teaspoon ground cumin
  1 clove of garlic, roughly chopped
  juice of 1 lemon
  salt and black pepper
  100g raw spinach or 100g roasted red peppers (optional
    if you want to try other flavours)

Tzatziki
  250g full-fat Greek yogurt
  1 cucumber, grated and squeezed to remove water
  2 tablespoons dried mint
  1 clove of garlic, finely grated
  black pepper

Crudités
  carrot sticks
  cucumber sticks
  celery sticks
  pepper sticks

246

sugar snap peas
radishes
cauliflower florets
broccoli florets

Other optional things to serve
salami
chorizo
sundried tomatoes
olives

For the butter bean hummus, place all the ingredients except for the seasoning into a mini chopper or food processor and blitz until smooth. Add salt and black pepper to taste and then transfer to a serving bowl.

If you fancy trying one of the other flavours, like spinach or red peppers, simply add that ingredient at the start along with all the other ingredients.

For the tzatziki, mix together all the ingredients in a mixing bowl and then season to taste with black pepper. Don't use salt in this as it will make the cucumber lose more water, making for a wet tzatziki. Transfer to a serving bowl.

Keep the dips in the fridge until needed.

Serve the dips alongside a mixed selection of crunchy raw veg, antipasti meats (optional if you'd prefer to keep this dish vegetarian), sundried tomatoes and olives.

TIP

If you are short on time, you can use shop-bought hummus and tzatziki, which will cut the prep time down to the time it takes to prepare the vegetables – no more than 5 minutes.

VEGETABLE TIKKA MASALA
WITH CAULIFLOWER RICE

batch cook / freezes well / vegetarian / vegan option

Serves 6

Takes 2 hours

Hands-on: 15 minutes / Hands-off: 1¾ hours

For the curry

- 1 tablespoon ghee (or 1 tablespoon olive oil for a vegan option)
- 1 celeriac, peeled and diced into 2cm chunks
- 2 aubergines, diced into 2cm chunks
- 2 onions, diced
- 3 red peppers, deseeded and diced into 2cm chunks
- 3 tablespoons tikka masala paste (with no added sugar or preservatives)
- 400g tin of plum or chopped tomatoes
- 400ml tin of coconut milk (look for a high percentage of coconut solids with no additives)
- 160ml coconut cream (check the labelling for any dubious ingredients)
- 400g tin of chickpeas, drained and rinsed
- 2 tablespoons chopped fresh coriander
- black pepper

For the cauliflower rice

- 1 tablespoon ghee (or 1 tablespoon olive oil for a vegan option)

1 cauliflower, blitzed or roughly chopped to resemble grains of rice (or pre-prepared cauliflower rice – best bought frozen and stored in the freezer until needed)

To make the curry, heat the ghee (or olive oil) in a large casserole pot. Add the celeriac, aubergine and onion. Cook on a high heat for 10–15 minutes until the aubergine has really started to soften and the celeriac has taken on some colour.

Add the peppers and tikka masala paste and stir to coat the rest of the vegetables. Reduce the heat and add the tomatoes, breaking them up with a wooden spoon (if using whole tinned tomatoes), and then the coconut milk and cream.

Add the chickpeas, stir to mix in, then allow the curry to come up to the boil, before turning the heat down and leaving it to gently simmer for 1½ hours, stirring occasionally to stop anything sticking.

After this time you should have perfectly cooked, soft celeriac and a thick, rich sauce. If you like it thicker, cook for another 10 minutes or so. Turn off the heat and add the coriander and some black pepper. Keep to one side.

To make the cauliflower rice, heat the ghee (or olive oil) in a large frying pan, then add the cauliflower. Cook on a high heat for 2–3 minutes until golden. The cauliflower rice can be served simply as it is, or you might like to add some extra coriander and a pinch of turmeric; or fry up some chopped mushrooms or even add some desiccated coconut, depending on what flavours you fancy.

AUBERGINE PARMIGIANA OR LASAGNE-ISH

batch cook / freezes well / vegetarian option

Serves 6
Takes 1 ½ hours
Hands-on: 30 minutes / Hands-off: 1 hour

  2 tablespoons olive oil
  1 large onion, diced
  4 celery stalks, diced
  500g minced beef (optional)
  2 tablespoons tomato purée
  680g passata
  1 tablespoon mixed herbs
  1 tablespoon dried oregano
  1 tablespoon red wine vinegar
  2 large aubergines, cut into 1.5 cm rounds
  olive oil, for brushing
  3 × 125g mozzarella balls
  25g basil leaves
  100g Parmesan, grated
  salt and black pepper

Heat the olive oil in a large saucepan or deep-sided frying pan and then add the onion and celery. Cook for 5 minutes to start to soften.

Add the beef if you are using it and break up with a wooden spoon. Cook for 5 minutes until you have no red meat left.

If you are not using the beef, then skip straight to adding the tomato purée.

Add the tomato purée and cook for a minute, stirring to coat everything in the pan. Add the passata, herbs and vinegar and some seasoning. Bring up to a boil and then reduce the heat and simmer for 40–50 minutes until you have a thickened sauce.

While the tomato sauce is cooking, heat a large frying pan. Brush a little olive oil over one side of the aubergine rounds and place them in a single layer in the hot pan. You will probably need to cook these in two or three batches. Leave to cook for 4–5 minutes, and once they are a deep golden brown, flip and cook for another 4–5 minutes until the other side is equally golden and the flesh has really started to soften. Remove to a plate and repeat for the remaining aubergine slices.

Tear the mozzarella on to some kitchen towel and pat it with another piece – this is just to remove any excess moisture as you don't want a really wet Parmigiana.

Preheat the oven to 190°C/170°C fan/gas 5.

Once the sauce has thickened, remove from the heat, take a large roasting dish and spread out a third of the sauce to coat the bottom. Add half the aubergine rounds in a layer, then add a good handful of basil leaves, some of the mozzarella and a sprinkle of Parmesan.

Repeat this with the next third of sauce, the rest of the aubergine, and so on. Finally, top the dish with the remaining sauce. Add the last of the basil, mozzarella and the rest of the Parmesan.

Place the roasting dish on to a foil-lined baking sheet (this is just to catch any of the bubbly juices as it cooks) and cook in the oven for 25–30 minutes until the cheese is golden and everything is bubbling.

Serve with a crisp green salad or with some steamed greens.

TIP

This dish is great to have as leftovers for another meal, either cold or reheated.

TOFU AND MIXED VEGETABLE STIR-FRY

vegan

Serves 2
Takes 30 minutes
Hands-on: 20 minutes / Hands-off: 10 minutes

  280g extra-firm tofu
  2 tablespoons extra virgin olive oil, plus extra to drizzle
  4 cloves of garlic, grated
  5 cm piece of ginger, peeled and grated
  2 red chillies, thinly sliced
  2 peppers, deseeded and cut into lengths
  100g green beans, top and tailed
  2 pak choi, sliced
  1 large carrot, peeled into ribbons
  1 courgette, peeled into ribbons
  150g beansprouts
  50g cashew nuts, roughly chopped
  2 tablespoons chopped coriander

Cut the tofu into 1cm fingers and then place on a piece of kitchen towel. Place another piece of kitchen towel on top and then place a chopping board on top of that with a couple of tins on top. You want to gently press any extra moisture out of the tofu as this will help it crisp up. Leave for 10 minutes and then place a wok on a high heat and pour in the extra virgin olive oil.

Add the strips of tofu and cook for 2–3 minutes each side until golden and crisp. Remove and place on a clean, dry piece of kitchen towel.

Pour in another splash of oil if needed and then add the garlic, ginger and chilli. Cook for 30 seconds until fragrant and then add the peppers and green beans. Cook for 4–5 minutes, tossing everything frequently, then add the white stalk of the pak choi and cook for another minute.

Lastly, add the carrot, courgette ribbons, beansprouts and pak choi leaves. Cook for another 2–3 minutes until the veg is just softening but still crisp and crunchy, then add the tofu back into the pan.

Divide between two serving plates, scatter over the cashew nuts and coriander and finish with a drizzle of extra virgin olive oil.

TIPS

Many supermarkets sell bags of ready-prepared vegetables for stir-fries, containing nothing but the veg, which would work well for this dish and save on time.

To bring out the natural oils of the nuts – for even more flavour – you can roast the cashews before using. To do this, spread out on a baking tray and roast in a warm oven (170°C/150°C fan/gas 3) for 10–15 minutes, shaking the tray every few minutes. Keep a close eye as the nuts can catch easily.

CRISPY BAKED CHICKEN
WITH CELERIAC CHIPS

Serves 2
Takes 1 hour
Hands-on: 10 minutes / Hands-off: 45–50 minutes

For the celeriac chips
  1 large celeriac, peeled and cut into 2cm wide chips
  2 tablespoons olive oil
  salt and black pepper

For the almond spice mix
  80g ground almonds
  20g ground flaxseed
  2 teaspoons smoked paprika
  ½ teaspoon cayenne pepper
  1 tablespoon dried oregano
  1 teaspoon dried thyme
  1 teaspoon garlic granules
  1 teaspoon onion powder
  salt and black pepper

For the chicken
  2 eggs
  6 pieces of skin-on chicken leg (e.g. 2 thighs, 4
    drumsticks)
  olive oil, for drizzling

Preheat the oven to 210°C/190°C fan/gas 7 and line two baking sheets with baking paper.

Place the celeriac chips into a large saucepan filled with water and bring to a boil. Keep at a simmer for 6 minutes, then drain and steam dry. Tip the chips on to one of the trays, drizzle over the olive oil and season generously. Keep to one side.

In a shallow bowl, mix together the almond spice mix ingredients with a pinch of salt and some black pepper.

Crack the eggs into another shallow dish and beat with a fork.

Take each piece of chicken and roll in the egg. Shake off any excess and then dip and roll in the almond spice mix. Put on to the second baking sheet and then repeat with all the remaining chicken.

Drizzle lightly with olive oil and then place both trays – one with the chicken and one with the chips – into the hot oven for 45–50 minutes. Remove the celeriac chips after 25 minutes and turn them, then return for the remaining 20–25 minutes.

When the celeriac chips are cooked through and golden brown and the chicken has formed a great crunchy crust, remove the trays from the oven. Delicious served with some green salad leaves or any Programme vegetables of your choosing.

CAULIFLOWER CHEESE

batch cook / freezes well / vegetarian

Serves 4
Takes 1 hour
Hands-on: 30 minutes / Hands-off: 30 minutes

1 large cauliflower (approx. 600g trimmed florets)
1 tablespoon olive oil
50g butter
50g arrowroot
¼ teaspoon ground nutmeg
1–2 teaspoons chipotle or regular chilli flakes (depending
   on preference and availability)
500ml whole milk
200g mature Cheddar, grated
150g creamy hard cheese, like Lancashire or Wensleydale,
   grated
2 tablespoons sunflower seeds
2 tablespoons pumpkin seeds
20g Parmesan, grated
salt and black pepper

Preheat the oven to 180°C/160°C fan/gas 4.

Place the cauliflower florets into a medium roasting dish
and drizzle over the olive oil. Toss to coat and then pop into
the oven for 30 minutes. Turn the florets every 10 minutes to
make sure they cook evenly.

While the cauliflower is cooking, melt the butter together with the arrowroot until well combined and it starts to foam. Add the nutmeg and chilli flakes (if using) and stir to combine. At this point, using a balloon whisk, start to slowly add the milk, little by little, whisking continuously until it is incorporated.

Once all the milk is in, turn off the heat and add the cheese. Allow the heat of the sauce to melt the cheese. Season with a little pinch of salt and lots of pepper.

When the cauliflower is cooked, add to the cheese sauce and stir to coat before pouring back into the roasting dish. Keep to one side.

Put the two types of seeds into a mini chopper and pulse until roughly chopped, or bash in a pestle and mortar. Stir through the Parmesan and then sprinkle all over the top of the cauliflower in the dish.

Increase the heat of the oven to 200°C/180°C fan/gas 6 and put the cauliflower cheese in. Bake for 20–25 minutes until a lovely golden brown and bubbling.

Serve with a green leaf salad or some steamed greens.

TIP

Arrowroot is a great alternative to other thickening agents. It contains more fibre than flour or cornstarch and will last a long time in your store cupboard.

NUT ROAST

vegetarian / great portable option

Serves 4
Takes 1½ hours
Hands-on: 30 minutes / Hands-off: 1 hour

2 tablespoons olive oil, plus extra to drizzle
1 red onion, diced
2 celery stalks, diced
1 red pepper, deseeded and diced
1 large carrot, peeled and diced
250g chestnut mushrooms (or mushroom of choice),
    diced
4 cloves of garlic, finely grated
150g dried red lentils
2 tablespoons tomato purée
1 tablespoon dried oregano
2 teaspoons smoked paprika
160g mixed nuts (like Brazil nuts, walnuts, almonds,
    pecans), chopped
3 large eggs, beaten
150g extra-mature Cheddar, grated
2 tablespoons chopped parsley
60g watercress and rocket salad
200g cherry tomatoes, halved
a drizzle of red wine vinegar
salt and black pepper

Preheat the oven to 180°C/160°C fan and line a medium roasting dish with non-stick baking paper.

Heat the olive oil in a large, deep-sided frying pan or wok and add the onion, celery, pepper and carrot and cook for 2–3 minutes. Then add the mushrooms and cook for another 12–15 minutes until they have softened and moisture from the mushrooms has stopped being released. Stir frequently to make sure it's cooking evenly.

Stir the garlic into the mix and cook for another 30 seconds, followed by the lentils and tomato purée. Stir well to combine and cook for 2 minutes before adding 325ml cold water.

Add the oregano, paprika and mixed nuts. Cook for no more than 5 minutes until the water has largely been absorbed by the lentils.

Turn off the heat and add the beaten eggs, Cheddar, parsley and some seasoning.

Once everything has been mixed together really well, pour it all into the lined roasting dish. Level off with the back of a spoon and cover with tin foil. Bake in the oven, covered, for 30 minutes, then remove the foil and bake for another 30–40 minutes until the nut roast has dried out, firmed up and started to go a deep golden brown round the edges.

Remove from the oven and allow to rest for 5 minutes to firm up before serving.

Serve alongside a salad of peppery leaves like watercress and rocket, with cherry tomatoes for freshness and a drizzle of olive oil and red wine vinegar.

FISH PIE WITH CELERIAC MASH

batch cook

Serves 6
Takes 1½ hours
Hands-on: 1 hour / Hands-off: 30 minutes

For the celeriac mash topping
    2 celeriac (approx. 900g peeled weight), peeled and diced
    60g butter
    1 tablespoon olive oil
    1 large onion, diced
    1 large leek, sliced in half lengthways and then sliced
    500ml whole milk
    2 bay leaves

For the fish pie filling
    400g cod loin
    200g undyed smoked haddock fillet
    200g salmon fillet
    150g raw king prawns
    or
    950g frozen fish pie mix

For the fish pie white sauce
    3 tablespoons arrowroot
    3 tablespoons chopped dill
    3 tablespoons chopped parsley
    zest of 1 lemon

150ml double cream
salt and black pepper

Preheat the oven to 190°C/170°C fan/gas 5.

Put the celeriac into a large saucepan, cover with cold water and place on a high heat. Bring to the boil and cook for 25 minutes or until tender all the way through.

While the celeriac is cooking, melt half the butter with the olive oil in a large frying pan and add the onion and leek. Cook gently for 10 minutes until softened and just starting to go golden.

While the onion and leek are cooking, place the milk and bay leaves into a high-sided pan and bring to a simmer. Add all the fish and prawns and poach for 4–5 minutes until just cooked. If you are using a frozen fish pie mix, cook according to the packet instructions. Use a slotted spoon to lift out the fish and keep to one side.

Add the arrowroot to the onion mix and stir well. Slowly add the poaching milk to start to make a white sauce. Keep stirring and adding in increments until all the milk is in. Cook for a few minutes until the sauce thickens.

Turn off the heat and add in the fish, dill, parsley, lemon zest and cream. Gently mix until everything is combined. Transfer to a large ovenproof dish.

Drain the celeriac and mash with the remaining butter and season to taste. Place back on the heat and stir continuously for a couple of minutes to help dry out the mash. You don't want a soggy fish pie.

Carefully spoon the celeriac on to the fish mix and use a fork to spread it out to cover the pie.

Bake in the hot oven for 25 minutes until golden and bubbling. Delicious served with greens like peas and green beans.

TIP

This is great to batch cook and freeze leftover portions. Defrost in the fridge overnight and reheat thoroughly in the oven until hot.

GRILLED CHICKEN BREAST WITH
SATAY SAUCE AND STIR-FRIED GREENS

Serves 2
Takes 25 minutes
Hands-on: 10 minutes / Hands-off: 15 minutes

For the satay sauce
    180ml coconut cream (check the labelling for any
      dubious ingredients)
    20g crunchy peanut butter (check there is no added
      sugar)
    juice of 1 large lime
    1 teaspoon soy sauce
    1 teaspoon chilli flakes

For the chicken
    2 chicken breasts, skin on
    3 tablespoons extra virgin olive oil
    200g Tenderstem broccoli
    350g spring greens, shredded
    1 teaspoon garlic granules
    1 teaspoon sesame seeds
    black pepper

Preheat the grill to its highest setting and line a baking sheet
with tin foil.

    Start by making the satay sauce. Whisk together the coconut cream and peanut butter in a mixing bowl and then add the lime juice, soy sauce and chilli flakes. Once all combined, keep to one side until needed.

Take a large piece of baking paper and place one of the chicken breasts on it. Fold the paper over and use a rolling pin to flatten it out to around 1.5cm thickness. Keep to one side and repeat with the other breast. Discard the baking paper.

Place the chicken on the baking sheet, drizzle over 1 tablespoon of the extra virgin olive oil and season with black pepper. Put the chicken under the grill for 8 minutes, then turn and cook for another 8 minutes.

While the chicken is cooking, heat the remaining extra virgin olive oil in a wok (or large frying pan) and add the broccoli. Toss to cook for 2 minutes, then add 80ml water and pop a lid over it to semi-steam cook for 5 minutes. Remove the lid, add the spring greens, garlic and sesame seeds and cook altogether until the greens have just wilted.

Remove the chicken, allow to rest for a couple of minutes and then slice. Drizzle over the satay sauce and serve alongside the greens.

TIPS

This also works really well with salmon. Grill the salmon for 12–15 minutes until it just starts to take on some colour and follow the rest of the recipe as is.

To use up leftover juiced lime halves, peel the lime before juicing and dry the peel, which can then be used as a garnish on a meal or infused with hot water as a herbal tea.

BRAISED COD WITH LETTUCE, PEAS AND CRÈME FRAÎCHE

Serves 2

Takes 15 minutes

Hands-on: 10 minutes / Hands-off: 5 minutes

1 tablespoon olive oil
20g butter
2 little gem lettuces, cut in half through the stalk
200g frozen peas
2 skinless cod fillets (approx. 150g each), fresh or frozen
3 tablespoons full-fat crème fraîche
1 tablespoon chopped parsley
juice of ½ lemon
salt and black pepper

Heat the olive oil and butter in a large frying pan over a gentle heat and then place in the four halves of lettuce, cut side down. Cook for 2 minutes and then add the frozen peas.

Cook the lettuce and peas for another 4 minutes and then make space for the two cod fillets. If you are using frozen fillets, check the packet instructions as you may need to increase the cooking time slightly. Cook for just a minute before adding the crème fraîche. Gently swirl the pan to help the crème fraîche melt into the butter and emulsify into a sauce.

After 3 minutes, flip the fish and the lettuce halves and cook the other side for 2–3 minutes, until the fish is just cooked. It should be opaque all the way through and wanting to just flake apart.

Once done, add the parsley, lemon juice and seasoning. Swirl to combine and then serve immediately.

CALAMARI WITH TARTARE SAUCE

Serves 2
Takes 20 minutes
Hands-on: 15 minutes / Hands-off: 5 minutes

For the tartare sauce
  2 tablespoons full-fat mayonnaise
  2 tablespoons full-fat Greek yogurt
  1 tablespoon capers, drained, rinsed and chopped
  2 gherkins, finely chopped
  ¼ teaspoon ground turmeric
  1 tablespoon finely chopped parsley
  zest and juice of 1 lemon, to taste
  salt and black pepper

For the calamari
  400g squid tubes, fresh or frozen and defrosted, cut into
      1.5cm rounds
  1 large egg, beaten
  100g ground almonds
  1 teaspoon paprika
  1 teaspoon garlic granules
  olive oil, for frying
  salt and black pepper

To serve
  lemon wedges

Start by making your tartare sauce. Place the mayonnaise, yogurt, capers, gherkins, turmeric and parsley into a small bowl and stir to mix. Add the lemon zest, some salt and pepper and as much lemon juice as you like. Keep to one side.

Take the squid and, if defrosted from frozen, pat it as dry as you can with some kitchen towel.

Place the beaten egg in one shallow dish, and the almonds, paprika, garlic and some seasoning in another.

Take the squid rings and dip them into the egg, then carefully toss in the almond mix to coat. Keep to one side while you heat around a centimetre of oil in a frying pan over a medium heat and then, very carefully, place the calamari into the pan in a single layer. Don't overcrowd the pan and unless you have a very large pan, it's probably best to do it in a few batches.

Cook the squid for a minute until the almonds go a light gold and then turn and cook the other side.

Remove from the oil with a slotted spoon and place on some kitchen paper to soak up the excess oil. Repeat for the other squid rings and then serve the calamari alongside the tartare sauce, with a big wedge of lemon.

These go brilliantly with some peppers and courgettes oven-roasted in a little olive oil with a pinch of dried oregano and seasoning for 20–25 minutes at 200°C/180°C fan/gas 6.

TIP

Leftover jarred capers can be used to accompany smoked salmon with some lemon and cream cheese or scattered in a salad.

LAMB AND HALLOUMI KEBABS
WITH ROCKET AND A YOGURT
AND MINT DRESSING

Serves 2
Takes 20 minutes, plus marinating
Hands-on: 5 minutes / Hands-off: 15 minutes

For the kebabs
    400g diced lamb
    200g halloumi cheese, cut into 3cm chunks
    1 red pepper, deseeded and cut into 3cm chunks
    1 red onion, cut into wedges
    1 tablespoon olive oil
    1 tablespoon dried oregano
    2 teaspoons dried mint
    ½ teaspoon garlic granules
    zest of 1 lemon

For the salad
    100g rocket leaves
    2 tablespoons full-fat yogurt
    juice of ½ lemon
    1 tablespoon chopped mint
    salt and black pepper

Place the lamb, halloumi, pepper, onion, olive oil, oregano, mint, garlic granules and lemon zest into a large mixing bowl and toss until everything is well coated. Cover, place in the fridge and leave to marinate for at least an hour (or overnight if that's easier).

When you are ready to eat, put your grill on the highest setting and thread four metal skewers with an equal mix of all the ingredients.

When the grill is really hot, place the kebabs underneath, quite close to the heat, and cook for 15–20 minutes until the lamb is cooked through, parts of the halloumi are golden brown and crisp and the pepper and onion are softening. Turn every 5 minutes or so to keep it cooking evenly.

Divide the rocket between two plates. Mix together the yogurt, lemon juice and mint, drizzle over the leaves and then top with two of the kebabs. Season with a little salt and pepper, to taste.

RECIPES

ROAST CHICKEN AND
VEGETABLE TRAYBAKE

Serves 2
Takes 1¼ hours
Hands-on: 15 minutes / Hands-off: 1 hour

4 skin-on and bone-in chicken thighs
2 peppers (red/yellow/orange), deseeded and cut into
   chunks
2 red onions, each cut into 8 wedges
1 aubergine, peeled and cut into chunks
1 large courgette, cut into chunks
6 cloves of garlic, skin on
1 tablespoon olive oil
1 teaspoon dried thyme
½ teaspoon smoked paprika
½ teaspoon chipotle or regular chilli flakes (depending
   on preference and availability)
½ teaspoon garlic granules
1 tablespoon red wine vinegar
1 tablespoon lemon thyme leaves or regular thyme
   (depending on preference and availability)
salt and black pepper

Preheat the oven to 200°C/180°C fan/gas 6.

Season the chicken with salt and pepper and then place the
thighs into a hot frying pan, skin side down, and cook for 10
minutes on low heat. This will start the fat rendering and will

help the skin to crisp up. By the time the 10 minutes are up, the skin should be a lovely pale gold, which will then only get better in the oven.

Remove from the heat and keep to one side.

Place the peppers, onion, aubergine, courgette and garlic cloves into a large roasting dish. Drizzle over the olive oil and sprinkle over the dried thyme, paprika, chilli flakes (if using) and garlic granules. Toss to coat everything, then nestle the thighs into the veg and drizzle the rendered fat over the veg.

Pop the dish into the oven and roast for 25 minutes, then remove the dish, turn the veg and roast for another 25 minutes.

Once the veg is tender and the chicken cooked all the way through, remove the dish from the oven, drizzle over the vinegar and sprinkle over the fresh lemon thyme.

Delicious as it is or cold with salad if you have leftovers.

TIP

You can also add 150g of sliced chorizo to the roasting dish for a little extra spice. For a vegetarian option, simply omit all the meat and increase the veg accordingly.

CHILLI CON CARNE WITH CHEDDAR, AVOCADO AND SOUR CREAM

batch cook / freezes well

Serves 6

Takes 2 hours

Hands-on: 30 minutes / Hands-off: 1 ½ hour

For the chilli
- 2 tablespoons olive oil
- 1 large red onion, diced
- 1 red pepper, deseeded and diced
- 3 celery stalks, diced
- 1 large courgette, grated
- 3 cloves of garlic, grated
- 2 tablespoons tomato purée
- 2 tablespoons dried oregano
- 1–2 teaspoons chilli powder (depending on preference)
- 1 teaspoon ground cumin
- 1 teaspoon ground coriander
- 750g minced beef
- 400g tin of chopped tomatoes
- 300ml beef stock
- 20g coriander, chopped
- salt and black pepper

For the toppings
- 120g Cheddar, grated

3 avocados, sliced
6 tablespoons sour cream

Heat the olive oil in a large frying pan and add the onion, pepper, celery, courgette and garlic and stir well to combine. Cook for 10 minutes, stirring frequently until everything has softened and just started to take on some colour.

Add the tomato purée and oregano and cook for another 2 minutes.

Add the chilli, cumin, coriander and beef mince. Stir well and break up the mince with your spoon. Turn the heat up high so you seal the meat, but be careful not to boil it.

Once there is no pink meat left, add the tomatoes and stir into the mix, followed by the stock and some seasoning. Stir and then once it is back to bubbling, reduce the heat to a simmer and cook for 1½ hours, stirring every 15 minutes or so to stop anything catching on the bottom of your pan.

By the end of the cooking time, the chilli should have thickened nicely. If you like it thicker, cook for another 10–15 minutes. Stir in the fresh coriander and then take off the heat.

Serve hot with some grated cheese, sliced avocado and a dollop of sour cream.

Steamed broccoli is also a great accompaniment to this dish.

TIP

This recipe is great for batch cooking. Extra chilli can be cooled and frozen for an easy meal another day.

BOLOGNESE AND COURGETTI

batch cook / freezes well

Serves 6
Takes 1½ hours
Hands-on: 30 minutes / Hands-off: 1 hour

2 tablespoons olive oil
1 large onion, diced
2 large carrots, peeled and diced
3 celery stalks, diced
4 cloves of garlic, grated
2 tablespoons tomato purée
1 tablespoon dried oregano
½ teaspoon ground nutmeg
750g minced beef
3 bay leaves
2 × 400g tins of plum or chopped tomatoes
1 tablespoon red wine vinegar
100ml whole milk
20g basil, roughly chopped
salt and black pepper

For the courgetti
6 courgettes, julienned or spiralized (or a pre-prepared
packet of courgetti)

To serve
Parmesan, grated

Heat the olive oil in a large saucepan and add the onion, carrot, celery and garlic. Cook over a medium heat for 10–15 minutes until everything has really softened and started to go golden. You need to stir fairly regularly to keep it all cooking evenly.

Once soft and golden, add the tomato purée, oregano and nutmeg, stir to combine and cook for another couple of minutes. Add the mince and use your spoon to help break it up. Turn the heat up as you want to seal the mince, but don't allow it to stew.

Once it is sealed (not red anymore) and sizzling away nicely, add the bay leaves, tinned tomatoes and red wine vinegar. Use your spoon to break up the tomatoes (if using whole tinned tomatoes). Bring up to a simmer and then reduce the heat.

Add the milk and mix well. Reduce the heat and simmer for 1 hour until thickened to your liking and then remove from the heat. Add the basil, season to taste and keep to one side.

Set up a saucepan and steamer basket. Bring a couple of centimetres of water to the boil so the basket is full of steam and add the courgetti. Cook for 1½ minutes then transfer to a colander and allow to steam-dry a little.

Serve the courgetti with the Bolognese and top with a sprinkle of Parmesan.

DARK CHOCOLATE TRUFFLES

Makes 40ish (one serving is 2)
Takes 20 minutes, plus chilling and shaping time
Hands-on: 15 minutes / Hands-off: 5 minutes

  300g dark chocolate, at least 85–90% cocoa solids, finely
    chopped
  300ml double cream
  70g unsalted butter
  3 tablespoons cocoa powder (unsweetened)

Place the finely chopped chocolate into a large mixing bowl.
Place the double cream and butter in a saucepan.

Put the saucepan on a gentle heat to melt the butter and
warm the cream. You don't want this to boil or steam, just be
warmed through.

Pour the cream mix over the chocolate and with a spatula
very gently stir it around the chopped chocolate. Leave to
stand and melt for 2 minutes and then gently stir together.
If the cream is too hot it can make the chocolate seize, but a
splash of cold whole milk can help bring it all back together
if needed.

Once you have a melted, glossy mix, cover and chill in the
fridge until firm. This will be a minimum of 2 hours. Then
remove from the fridge and let stand for 10–20 minutes to
just start to warm up.

Sieve the cocoa into a shallow dish.

Take heaped teaspoons of the chocolate mix and shape

quickly with your hands into round balls. Drop them into the cocoa and roll to coat. Transfer to a storage container as you go.

Keep the truffles in the fridge. They should last for a few weeks.

DARK CHOCOLATE
PEANUT BUTTER BALLS

vegan

Makes 12 (one serving is 2)
Takes 15 minutes, plus chilling
Hands-on: 10 minutes / Hands-off: 5 minutes

    150g peanut butter, smooth or crunchy depending
       on your preference, or another nut butter of your
       choosing, e.g. almond butter
    50–100g ground almonds
    100g dark chocolate, at least 85–90% cocoa solids
    a pinch of sea salt (optional)

Place the nut butter and 50g of almonds into a bowl. Use a spoon to mix the two together. How much additional ground almond you need depends on how loose or oily your nut butter is (some are firm and won't need any extra, some are looser and will take all the extra). You need the mix not to be oily so that it holds a round shape when you form it into balls, so add more ground almond if needed.

Once you have the right consistency, shape into 12 balls and pop them on to a baking sheet lined with non-stick baking paper and then into the fridge.

Place the chocolate into a mixing bowl and melt either in the microwave in 20-second bursts or over a little pan of boiling water, as a bain-marie.

Once the chocolate has melted, remove the peanut butter

balls from the fridge and one by one stab them with a tooth-pick and dip into the chocolate. Alternatively, spoon the melted chocolate over the peanut butter balls. Place them back on to the non-stick baking paper, add a pinch of sea salt to each if using, and then chill in the fridge until set.

You can store these in the fridge for a few weeks.

FRUITY FROGURT

Ready in under 15

Serves 2
Takes 5 minutes

  200g full-fat Greek yogurt
  75g frozen berries (raspberries/strawberries/
    blackberries)
  2 squares of 85% or 90% dark chocolate, roughly chopped
  2 teaspoons roasted hazelnuts, chopped

Place the yogurt and frozen berries into a mini chopper or food processor and quickly pulse together to just break up the fruit a little and combine into the yogurt. The frozen berries will chill the yogurt to give it a sorbet consistency.

Divide between two serving bowls and sprinkle over the chocolate and hazelnuts. Eat immediately.

Alternatively, you can pulse the yogurt and fruit, transfer to a container suitable for the freezer, and freeze for a couple of hours if you want more of an ice cream feel.

TIPS

  If you are freezing the frogurt, freeze a couple of hours before you want to eat it – don't leave it in the freezer for too long otherwise ice crystals will form.

  Roasted hazelnuts (with no other dubious ingredients) tend to be widely available in the baking section of most supermarkets.

Super-speedy recipes:
your Programme 'convenience food'

The challenge that I set myself when writing these super-speedy recipes for you is that I needed to be able to describe their preparation in no more than three sentences. As it turns out, this proved to be more than enough! We are all busy and some days you could be feeling particularly short of time. This means that your Programme 'convenience food' needs to be as quick and easy as the food industry's 'inconvenience food'. The beauty of these ideas is their conjuring trick of being super-speedy and simple yet also delicious and satisfying – the food of Programme champions.

Super-speedy ideas

All servings are for one (unless otherwise stated). Increase as you need, depending on how many people you are eating with. You can serve with any Programme veg of your choosing.

Boiled eggs
Add 2 eggs to a pan of boiling water and cook for 5 minutes for soft-boiled (with a runny yolk) and 10 minutes for hard-boiled eggs.

Egg mayo
Add 2 eggs to a pan of boiling water and cook for 10 minutes. Place the pan in the sink and run under cold water for 20 seconds or so, before shelling the eggs under a running cold tap. Pat dry, mash through mayonnaise using a fork and season with salt and pepper.

Fried egg, spinach and ham stack
Arrange a couple of pieces of ham on a plate and top with a handful of spinach leaves. Fry 2 eggs in a pan with some olive oil or butter. Place the eggs directly on top of the spinach leaves to wilt them and season with salt and pepper.

Tuna mayo
Drain a tin of tuna and tip into a bowl. Using a fork, mash up the tuna with mayonnaise and season with salt and pepper.

Vinaigrette dressing – this is enough for two servings
Add 3 tablespoons olive oil, 1 tablespoon white wine vinegar, ½ teaspoon Dijon or wholegrain mustard, salt and pepper to a clean jam jar. Shake to combine.

Pear, blue cheese and walnut salad
Chop the pear into quarters and then quarter again and mix with green leaves – spinach works well. Crumble in blue cheese and walnuts. Goes well with the vinaigrette dressing.

Total salad

To a bowl, add any combination of salad leaves (like pak choi, lettuce, spinach leaves), red or green cabbage, peeled chopped carrots, celery, chopped tomatoes, chopped cucumber, nuts (e.g. toasted almonds or raw walnuts) and seeds (e.g. pumpkin or sunflower), sundried tomatoes, olives, chunks of Cheddar, feta (or other cheese). Dress with olive oil (or the vinaigrette dressing on the previous page) and season with salt and pepper.

Mozzarella and tomato salad with basil and olive oil

Slice the mozzarella and tomatoes into discs and arrange on a plate. Tear the basil leaves and place on top of the mozzarella and tomatoes. Drizzle with olive oil and season with salt and pepper.

Turkey or ham roll ups with sliced Cheddar and tomato

Stack the cheese on top of the turkey or ham and top with sliced tomato. Season with salt and pepper and roll up.

Smoked salmon roll ups with cream cheese

Spread the cream cheese on to the smoked salmon, season with black pepper and roll up. Good with a squeeze of lemon juice.

Chicken traybake

Place 2 chicken thighs (bone in, skin on) into a greased baking dish and shake over a powdered spice mix like jerk, piri piri or ras el hanout (check they contain no added sugar or other dubious ingredients). Add a glug of olive oil and shake the pan so that the oil coats the chicken. Season with salt and pepper and cook in a preheated oven (210°C/190°C fan/ gas 7) for 30 minutes or until the chicken is cooked through.

Oven-baked sausages (ensure the sausages have a high meat content – more than 90 per cent)

Oven bake or grill according to the instructions on the label.

Gammon steak

Grill according to the instructions on the label.

Lamb steak

Grill according to the instructions on the label.

Pan-fried steak

Take the steak out of the fridge 10 minutes before cooking so that it isn't fridge cold and pat dry with kitchen towel. Heat a heavy-based frying pan on a high heat on the hob until very hot but not smoking. Add the steak to the pan and cook for 2 minutes on each side for a medium-rare steak.

Grilled halloumi

Cut the halloumi into 1cm thick slices. Place under a hot grill for 4 minutes, turning the cheese halfway through.

Cauliflower mash – serves 4

Add florets from a whole cauliflower to a saucepan of boiling water and cook for 10 minutes or until tender (easily pierced with a fork), before draining using a colander or sieve and placing in a mixing bowl or the bowl of a food processor. Add butter, cream cheese or Cheddar (if wanted) and season with salt and pepper. Mash with a fork or masher or blitz until smooth in a food processor or with a stick blender.

Bun-less hamburgers or cheeseburgers

Shape minced beef into a burger patty and season with salt and pepper. Grill for approximately 8 minutes (depending on the thickness of your burger), turning halfway through. For a cheeseburger, top with cheese 1 minute before the end of the cooking time and return to the grill until melted.

Oven-baked salmon steaks

Preheat the oven to 180°C/160°C fan/gas 4. Season the salmon with salt and pepper, wrap loosely in tin foil and place in a baking tray. Cook for 15 minutes or until the fish looks opaque and flakes easily.

Roast chicken stuffed with onion and lemon – serves 4 to 6 depending on the size of the chicken

Chop a lemon in half and an onion in quarters and use to stuff the chicken cavity. Drizzle olive oil over the chicken skin and season with salt and pepper. Cook in a preheated oven (200°C/180°C fan/gas 6) for the time stated on the label (this will depend on the weight of the chicken).

Dark chocolate with nut butter

Spread a teaspoon or two of a nut butter, like peanut, hazelnut or almond butter, on to a few squares of dark chocolate about the size of a credit card. You can also sprinkle on some flaked sea salt crystals.

Strawberries and cream

Wash the strawberries, cut off the stalks and, depending on the size of the strawberries, cut in half or into quarters. Place in a bowl and pour over the cream. You can use single, double or clotted cream but please choose not to use the whipped cream in a can as this often contains added sugar.

Full-fat Greek yogurt with berries

Spoon the yogurt into a bowl and add berries of your choice, like strawberries, raspberries, blueberries or blackberries. Use frozen berries for a cooling alternative. You can also add nuts and/or seeds.

Sample Menu: One week of amazing Programme eating

Key: Bold: in main recipe section   Italics: in super-speedy ideas

	Monday	Tuesday	Wednesday	Thursday	Friday	Saturday	Sunday
First meal of the day – the time that you open your Eating Window	**Scrambled eggs with smoked salmon, mushrooms and spinach**	*Fried egg, spinach and ham stack*	*Full-fat Greek yogurt with berries*	*Over-baked sausages with raw spinach leaves drizzled with olive oil and garnished with pumpkin seeds*	*Grilled halloumi, cucumber and celery sticks* Handful of almonds	*Egg mayo with cucumber and celery sticks*	*Pear, blue cheese and walnut salad*
Second meal (lunch/dinner)	*Tuna mayo with carrot sticks and cherry tomatoes* Cheddar cheese Pear with a handful of Brazil nuts	*Bun-less cheeseburger with steamed broccoli florets* **One or two dark chocolate peanut butter balls**	**Feta and red onion egg muffins with a green salad** **One or two dark chocolate truffles**	*Total salad*	**Bolognese and courgetti**	*Turkey or ham roll ups with sliced Cheddar and tomato* Crudités with hummus *Strawberries and cream*	**Frittata with a green salad** *Dark chocolate and nut butter*
Final meal (dinner)	*Pan-fried steak with green beans* A few squares of dark chocolate – about the size of a credit card – with a cup of camomile tea	**Lamb and halloumi kebabs with rocket and a yogurt and mint dressing**	**Fish pie with celeriac mash**	**Braised cod with lettuce, peas and crème fraîche**	**Mezze platter** An apple with a couple of teaspoons of nut butter	**Thai cauliflower and coconut soup** **Fruity frogurt**	**Chilli con carne with Cheddar, avocado and sour cream** with steamed green beans

How to use your sample menu

This is a guide not a prescription!

The idea of the sample menu is simply to give you a feeling for what a week of delicious Programme eating could look like. You don't need to eat scrambled eggs on Monday and the mezze platter on Friday. Pick and choose the food that *you* like, *when* you like. You might want to do some mixing and matching, for example taking the celeriac chips from the crispy baked chicken recipe and enjoying them with your bun-less cheeseburger. You could also adapt some of your own favourite dishes, adjusting them so that they don't spike your blood sugar levels and require insulin (the fat controller) to come along sweeping into fat storage. For example, if you make a delicious lamb and potato curry with rice, you could substitute the potato for celeriac and the rice for cauliflower rice.

Why isn't there a meal called 'breakfast'?

You'll notice that I haven't called the first meal of the day breakfast. This is because when you get up and running with your Eating Window, you might find that you are not hungry first thing in the morning. You could instead end up first eating sometime between 11am and 2pm. This is around the time that most of my patients choose to open their Eating Window. So as to avoid any uncertainty about timings, I have called your first eating opportunity the first meal of the day, rather than breakfast.

How many meals a day?

As you can see, the sample menu includes three meals each day. This doesn't mean that you *have* to eat three meals a day. Remember that the Programme is about tuning in and listening to your body's messages. Of course, if your ghrelin hunger signal is strong three times a day, you should respond to that message and enjoy any delicious Programme food of your choosing. However, you are likely to find that when you eat in the Programme way, the fullness hormone text messages from your gut to your brain are now coming through loud and clear. Many of my patients love this sense of fullness, leaving them feeling satisfied and able to easily move on from food for several hours after eating. My patients also often find that eating three meals in an eight-hour open Eating Window just feels like too much food in that space of time. For both these reasons, once my patients hit their Programme stride, many choose to eat two meals a day or two meals, plus a third smaller something at another time.

Your Programme, your choices

Most importantly, this is your Programme, your way. So please do tailor both your timings and food choices to make them perfectly right for you, enjoying the full abundance, flavour and satisfaction of good eating in a life that is full of choices.

Notes for clinicians

Some notes to help clinicians support
their patients on The Full Diet

In my experience, almost everybody can benefit from The
Full Diet. Even my patients with very serious medical conditions have achieved significant weight-loss success, as well as
great improvements in their health and wellbeing. The Full
Diet is a story of a patient-clinician partnership, and while
every patient will benefit from your support and encouragement, there are certain people for whom your medical care
will be particularly valuable:

- When they start the Programme, **people with type
  2 diabetes** usually see their blood glucose quickly
  reduce to normal. This could cause hypoglycaemia if
  they continue to take glucose-lowering medications, so
  careful planning is needed:

  - To prevent hypoglycaemia, I stop sulphonylureas
    (like gliclazide) and I down-titrate insulin
    injections, guided by my patients' home blood
    glucose checks. To give you an idea of the rapidity
    of the Programme's glycaemic benefits, Anil, my

patient whose inspiring words open Chapter 1, completely stopped his insulin injections within 48 hours of starting the Programme. So vigilance and good lines of communication are really key, with many patients benefitting from using a continuous glucose monitoring system (CGMS) during this time.

- ○ Before beginning the Programme, I stop SGLT-2 inhibitors (like empagliflozin and dapagliflozin) because of the rare but reported risk of euglycemic ketoacidosis with this class of drug when carbohydrates are reduced.

- To prevent drug-induced hypotension, my patients taking **anti-hypertensive medication** use a home blood-pressure monitor to track the fall in their blood pressure. These readings guide my advice on anti-hypertensive dose reduction and de-prescribing.

- Eating more vitamin K-rich foods, like green leafy vegetables, can lead to INR instability in **patients taking warfarin**. Regular INR monitoring is essential to guide warfarin dose-titration.

- If your patient has a **compromised immune system**, some Programme food choices will need to be modified. For example, they should avoid foods like kefir that contain live cultures and cook red meat until it is well done. It is a good idea to communicate

with their specialist about these and other dietary
considerations.

- In the same way, if you have a patient who has a
  complex health background, it's always helpful to
  collaborate with their specialists, so that they can offer
  their support and give expert advice if needed.

- Some commentators have asked whether time-
  restricted eating could drive **disordered eating**. I
  have not found this in my practice. In fact, as reported
  in our research study, our patients' eating patterns
  improve in the Programme. As ever, a thorough
  clinical history is key, as well as a compassionate
  discussion and signposting of best next steps if eating
  issues are identified.

- As people lose weight on The Full Diet, those with
  sleep apnoea often find their overnight CPAP is not
  needed anymore. It's a good idea to arrange a sleep
  study to confirm this and then your patients will have
  the happy task of returning their CPAP machine to the
  hospital.

- As your patients' health and quality of life improve,
  some who take an **anti-depressant** will feel it is
  no longer required. Here, I arrange a mental health
  assessment and if your patient and the clinician

agree, then anti-depressants can be down-titrated and stopped.

- It's a good idea to track your patients' **blood tests** over time. This will support their clinical care and is also a major momentum boost when, for example, your patients with fatty liver hear their liver function tests are now normal and when people with diabetes or pre-diabetes learn that their HbA1c is now in the normal range.

As your patients progress through their Programme journey, I am sure you will find, as I have, great fulfilment in seeing their weight fall and their health improve, as well as the privilege of sharing in news of work promotions, new relationships, dreams fulfilled and opportunities taken.

Acknowledgements

Imperial-SatPro (as we call The Full Diet in our hospital) changes lives because science and medicine succeed through collaboration. If it takes a village to raise a child, then it takes the academic rigor and clinical talents of pioneering colleagues to build a weight-loss programme. I am grateful to the outstanding doctors, surgeons and scientists who co-authored the original I-SatPro research study: Dr Vicky Salem, Dr Haya Alessemii, Dr Samantha Scholtz, Dr Owais Dar, Dr Alex Miras, Professor Karim Meeran, Professor Sir Steve Bloom, Mr Ahmed Ahmed, Mr Sanjay Purkayastha, Dr Harvey Chahal and Professor Tricia Tan. Thanks must also go to the National Institute for Health Research (NIHR) and Imperial-Biomedical Research Centre (BRC) for their generous funding support.

I am lucky to work with and learn from friends and colleagues, past and present, at the Imperial Weight Centre, whose expertise and clinical brilliance make it such a centre of excellence: Consultant Endocrinologists: Dr Harvey Chahal, Dr Chioma Izzi-Engbeaya, Dr Alex Miras and Professor Tricia Tan; Consultant Surgeons: Mr Ahmed Ahmed, Mr Sherif Hakky, Mr Krishna Moorthy, Mr Sanjay Purkayastha and Mr Christos Tsironis; Consultant Anaesthetist and Clinical Service Lead: Dr Jonathan Cousins; Consultant

Anaesthetists: Dr Mike Kynoch and Dr Francesca Rubulotta; Consultant Gastroenterologist: Dr Devinder Bansi; Clinical Research Fellow: Dr Julia Kenkre; Consultant Psychiatrists: Dr Samantha Scholtz, Dr Angharad Ruttley and Dr Amrit Sachar; Specialist Psychologists: Dr Daniela Alves, Dr Kelly Buttigieg, Dr Athena Foran, Dr Meila Roy and Dr Michael Shankleman; Diabetes Nurse Specialist: Anna Sackey; Clinical Nurse Specialists: Karen O'Donnell, Louisa Brolly, Ciara Price and Lisa Rickers; and Specialist Dieticians: Candace Bovill-Taylor, Jo Boyle, Rhian Houghton, Kate Parry and Jess Upton. Sincere thanks also to our brilliant MDT co-ordinators, Debbie O'Rourke (Tier 4) and Sahra Jama (Tier 3) and the meticulous administrative support of Cathy Dolan, Khadra Hassan and Fatma Shalaby, as well as our super-managers, Tom Connolly, Izabela Dubas, Clare Flatters, Chris Hughes, Anna Kennedy and Charlotte Quigley.

At the Imperial Centre for Endocrinology, it is a joy to work with such smart and kind colleagues who have taught me what excellent patient care looks like: Professor Karim Meeran, Dr Anjali Amin, Dr Preeshila Behary, Dr Emma Hatfield, Dr Neil Hill, Dr Channa Jayasena, Dr Niamh Martin, Ms Debbie Peters, Professor Amir Sam, Dr George Tharakan, Dr Risheka Walls and Dr Florian Wernig. Thanks also to Mehveen Meheralli and Shameeca Wilson for their superb secretarial support.

I want to thank my brilliant, brave and clever friend Dr Vicky Salem, who is always so wise and generous, and Dr Haya Alessimii whose tireless, gentle care for our patients has been exceptional.

ACKNOWLEDGEMENTS

I have had the privilege to know and work with some of the greats of endocrinology: Professor Sir Steve Bloom who teaches what the best science looks like by example; Professor Waljit Dhillo whose leadership and support have been so important to my story; Dr James Gardiner for his expert PhD supervision and for patiently sharing the beauty of molecular biology with me. The Programme would not exist without the vision, generosity and academic expertise of Professor Tricia Tan who championed I-SatPro from the very beginning. I became an endocrinologist because of Professor Karim Meeran – I am so grateful for his mentorship, teaching and exceptional kindness over the past two decades. My colleagues and patients had said for years, 'You should write a book', but when Prof said, 'You should write a book' – I wrote a book. And as usual he was right.

I was very fortunate to be taught at Oxford by Professor John Morris whose methodical, questioning intellect showed me how to think about the human body; and Professor Jaideep Pandit whose sheer love of physiology was absolutely contagious. I have thought of Jaideep's tutorials throughout my career.

Many thanks go to the team at London Metabolic Laboratory, especially Dr Boon Lim, a Consultant Cardiologist who looks after hearts from the heart, and James Harwood for being a (top dog) friend as well as a compassionate and deeply knowledgeable Programme coach. Much gratitude also goes to Veronica Casian for bringing the sunshine with her and for the love and care she puts into everything she does, and

301

to Simona Vasile for her many years of kindness, help and
support.

Less than a year ago, I was a doctor who wanted to write
a book. My brilliant literary agent, Will Francis, made that
dream a reality. Many, many thanks to Will for his excellent
judgement, assured expertise, kindness, and belief in the
book from our very first meeting. Thanks also go to Will's
superb colleagues at Janklow & Nesbit: Ren Balcombe,
Megan Browne, Kirsty Gordon, Ellis Hazelgrove, Michael
Steger and Maimy Suleiman.

The Programme has found its natural home with the outstanding team at Penguin Michael Joseph. I owe so much
gratitude to my publisher Fenella Bates whose talent, experience and vision have given The Full Diet its wings – Fenella's
enthusiasm, warmth and gift for bringing out the best in
people make her an absolute joy to work with. Lots of thanks
also go to Paula Flanagan for her laser-sharp editing, as well
as her genius for getting things done. I am really grateful to
Helena Cauldon for her sparkling editing of the manuscript,
my copy-editor Kay Halsey for her meticulous eye for detail
and Emma Henderson who, as if by magic, seamlessly trans-
formed the manuscript from a collection of Word documents
into a real-life book. Gaby Young, Jen Harlow, Ali Nazari,
Vicky Photiou and Lucy Upton have been a powerhouse of
a publicity team – taking The Full Diet from a meeting room
at Hammersmith Hospital to a global audience. It has also
been such a pleasure to know and work with: Inês Cortesão,
Xanthea Johnston, Tim Lane, Jenna Sandford and Kallie
Townsend – very many thanks for all the good things that

you have brought to the book. The energy and creative vision of the wider team have also been so much fun to be part of: Will Bremridge, Will Carne, Nella Gocal and Kat Meade.

It was my brilliant, clever dad, Dr Khalid Hameed, who inspired me to be a doctor. His star quality of making it seem that the lights have been switched on wherever he is remains inimitable. So much of what I have achieved would not have been possible without my incredible mum, Christine Hameed – from teaching me to read, to cutting every medical article out of the newspapers in the year before my medical school interviews, to now being the most generous, helpful and loving Maa-Maa, thank you for it all. My love and thanks also go to my parents-in-law (and now super-grandparents), Lynn and Steve Greenwold, who I have known for more than half my life and who have always been such steadfast and loving supporters.

I have three great friends, who I am so proud to call my siblings, Hasan, Imran and Amna Hameed. I am also very lucky to be part of a huge and loving family, including: Ghazala Hameed, Sophia Javaid Hameed, Asad Khan, Reza Javaid, Alia Brahimi, Noor and Lara Hameed, Spencer Eade, Max, Natalie, Stella and Clara Eade and Michael and Tara Greenwold. I also owe so many thanks to my best friends, who are also my family, for a lifetime of love and happy times: Lauren Mishcon, Misha Moore, Vicky Salem, Elizabeth Lands, Mark Nichols, Fariha Sultan and all her beautiful family, and Farima and Duncan Perry.

The five greatest blessings in my life are Jonathan, Sibella, Teddy, Hal and Raphael Bear. I carry you in my heart, I am never without you. This book is dedicated to you, Jonathan.

It has only been possible, like everything good in life, because of your love and encouragement. You are my energy, my courage and my home.

And, finally, this Programme is about and for my patients – the stars of I-SatPro – whose pioneering spirit, generosity and courage have blazed a trail for so many others to now benefit from the Programme. Thank you. I have taught you the science of I-SatPro and you have taught me everything else about the Programme. It is the greatest privilege to know you and to share in your success.

References

Chapter 1: Food

Department for Environment, Food and Rural Affairs, 'Family food datasets Detailed annual statistics on family food and drink purchases', Published 13 December 2012; Last updated 16 November 2020. Available at: https://www.gov.uk/government/statistical-data-sets/family-food-datasets

Ebbeling CB, Knapp A, Johnson A, Wong JMW, Greco KF, Ma C, Mora S, Ludwig DS, 'Effects of a low-carbohydrate diet on insulin-resistant dyslipoproteinemia – a randomized controlled feeding trial', *Am J Clin Nutr.* 2021 Sep 28: nqab287. doi: 10.1093/ajcn/nqab287. Epub ahead of print.

Estruch R, Ros E, Salas-Salvadó J, Covas MI, Corella D, Arós F, Gómez-Gracia E, Ruiz-Gutiérrez V, Fiol M, Lapetra J, Lamuela-Raventos RM, Serra-Majem L, Pintó X, Basora J, Muñoz MA, Sorlí JV, Martinez JA, Fitó M, Gea A, Hernán MA, Martínez-González MA, PREDIMED Study Investigators, 'Primary Prevention of Cardiovascular Disease with a Mediterranean Diet Supplemented with Extra-Virgin Olive Oil or Nuts', *N Engl J Med.* 2018 Jun 21; 378 (25): e34.

Foster R and Lunn J, '40th Anniversary Briefing Paper: Food availability and our changing diet', *Nutrition Bulletin (British Nutrition Foundation)* 2007 Sep; 32 (3): 187–249.

Hameed S, Salem V, Alessimii H, Scholtz S, Dar O, Miras AD, Meeran K, Bloom SR, Ahmed AR, Purkayastha S, Chahal H, Tan

T, 'Imperial Satiety Protocol: A new non-surgical weight-loss programme, delivered in a health care setting, produces improved clinical outcomes for people with obesity', *Diabetes Obes Metab.* 2021 Jan 23 (1): 270–5.

Howard BV, Van Horn L, Hsia J, Manson JE, Stefanick ML, Wassertheil-Smoller S, Kuller LH, LaCroix AZ, Langer RD, Lasser NL, Lewis CE, Limacher MC, Margolis KL, Mysiw WJ, Ockene JK, Parker LM, Perri MG, Phillips L, Prentice RL, Robbins J, Rossouw JE, Sarto GE, Schatz IJ, Snetselaar LG, Stevens VJ, Tinker LF, Trevisan M, Vitolins MZ, Anderson GL, Assaf AR, Bassford T, Beresford SA, Black HR, Brunner RL, Brzyski RG, Caan B, Chlebowski RT, Gass M, Granek I, Greenland P, Hays J, Heber D, Heiss G, Hendrix SL, Hubbell FA, Johnson KC, Kotchen JM, 'Low-fat dietary pattern and risk of cardiovascular disease: the Women's Health Initiative Randomized Controlled Dietary Modification Trial', *JAMA* 2006 Feb 8; 295 (6): 655–66.

Ludwig DS, Aronne LJ, Astrup A, de Cabo R, Cantley LC, Friedman MI, Heymsfield SB, Johnson JD, King JC, Krauss RM, Lieberman DE, Taubes G, Volek JS, Westman EC, Willett WC, Yancy WS, Ebbeling CB, 'The carbohydrate-insulin model: a physiological perspective on the obesity pandemic', *Am J Clin Nutr.* 2021 Sep 13; 114 (6): 1873–85. Epub ahead of print.

Mozaffarian D and Ludwig DS, 'Dietary guidelines in the 21st century–a time for food', *JAMA* 2010 Aug 11; 304 (6): 681–2.

NHS Digital, 'Health Survey for England, 2019: Overweight and obesity in adults and children. Published 2020. Available at: https://files.digital.nhs.uk/9D/4195D5/HSE19-Overweight-obesity-rep.pdf

Nordmann AJ, Suter-Zimmermann K, Bucher HC, Shai I, Tuttle KR, Estruch R, Briel M, 'Meta-analysis comparing Mediterranean to low-fat diets for modification of cardiovascular risk factors', *Am J Med.* 2011 Sep; 124 (9): 841–51.e2.

Pang MD, Goossens GH, Blaak EE, 'The Impact of Artificial Sweeteners on Body Weight Control and Glucose Homeostasis', *Front Nutr.* 2021 Jan 7; 7: 598340.

Ramsden CE, Zamora D, Majchrzak-Hong S, Faurot KR, Broste SK, Frantz RP, Davis JM, Ringel A, Suchindran CM, Hibbeln JR, 'Re-evaluation of the traditional diet-heart hypothesis: analysis of recovered data from Minnesota Coronary Experiment (1968-73)', *BMJ* 2016 Apr 12; 353: i1246.

Rosenbaum S, Skinner RK, Knight IB, Garrow JS, 'A survey of heights and weights of adults in Great Britain, 1980', *Ann Hum Biol.* 1985 Mar–Apr 12 (2): 115–27.

Rupp R, 'The Butter Wars: When Margarine Was Pink', *National Geographic* 2014. Available at: https://www.nationalgeographic.com/culture/article/the-butter-wars-when-margarine-was-pink

Shai I, Schwarzfuchs D, Henkin Y, Shahar DR, Witkow S, Greenberg I, Golan R, Fraser D, Bolotin A, Vardi H, Tangi-Rozental O, Zuk-Ramot R, Sarusi B, Brickner D, Schwartz Z, Sheiner E, Marko R, Katorza E, Thiery J, Fiedler GM, Blüher M, Stumvoll M, Stampfer MJ, 'Dietary Intervention Randomized Controlled Trial (DIRECT) Group. Weight loss with a low-carbohydrate, Mediterranean, or low-fat diet', *N Engl J Med.* 2008 Jul 17; 359: 229–41.

Sylvetsky AC, Brown RJ, Blau JE, Walter M, Rother KI, 'Hormonal responses to non-nutritive sweeteners in water and diet soda', *Nutr Metab (Lond).* 2016 Oct 21; 13: 71.

United States Department of Health and Human Services and United States Department of Agriculture, '2015–2020 Dietary Guidelines for Americans', 8th Edition. December 2015. Available at: http://health.gov/dietaryguidelines/2015/guidelines

United States Senate, 'Dietary Guidelines for Americans: Hearing before a subcommittee of the committee on appropriations. United

States Senate. Ninety Sixth Congress, Second Session. Special Hearing Department of Agriculture. Department of Health and Human Services. Non-Departmental Witnesses', United States Government Printing Office: Washington 1980.

Unwin D, Haslam D, Livesey G, 'It is the glycaemic response to, not the carbohydrate content of food that matters in diabetes and obesity: The glycaemic index revisited', *Journal of Insulin Resistance* 2016 Aug 19; 1 (1): a8.

Wang QP, Simpson SJ, Herzog H, Neely GG, 'Chronic Sucralose or L-Glucose Ingestion Does Not Suppress Food Intake', *Cell Metab.* 2017 Aug 1; 26: 279–80.

Wasserman DH, 'Four grams of glucose', *Am J Physiol Endocrinol Metab.* 2009 Jan; 296 (1): E11–21.

Willett WC, Stampfer MJ, Manson JE, Colditz GA, Speizer FE, Rosner BA, Sampson LA, Hennekens CH, 'Intake of trans fatty acids and risk of coronary heart disease among women', *Lancet* 1993 Mar 6; 341(8845): 581–5.

Chapter 2: Gut–brain signals

Batterham RL, Cohen MA, Ellis SM, Le Roux CW, Withers DJ, Frost GS, Ghatei MA, Bloom SR, 'Inhibition of food intake in obese subjects by peptide YY3-36', *N Engl J Med.* 2003 Sep 4; 349 (10): 941–8.

Batterham RL, Cowley MA, Small CJ, Herzog H, Cohen MA, Dakin CL, Wren AM, Brynes AE, Low MJ, Ghatei MA, Cone RD, Bloom SR, 'Gut hormone PYY (3-36) physiologically inhibits food intake', *Nature* 2002 Aug 8; 418: 650–54.

Batterham RL, Heffron H, Kapoor S, Chivers JE, Chandarana K, Herzog H, Le Roux CW, Thomas EL, Bell JD, Withers DJ, 'Critical role for peptide YY in protein-mediated satiation and body-weight regulation', *Cell Metab.* 2006 Sep; 4 (3): 223–33.

Chandler-Laney PC, Morrison SA, Goree LL, Ellis AC, Casazza K, Desmond R, Gower BA, 'Return of hunger following a relatively high carbohydrate breakfast is associated with earlier recorded glucose peak and nadir', *Appetite* 2014 Sep; 80: 236–41.

Chaudhri OB, Salem V, Murphy KG, Bloom SR, 'Gastrointestinal satiety signals', *Annu Rev Physiol.* 2008; 70: 239–55.

Considine RV, Sinha MK, Heiman ML, Kriauciunas A, Stephens TW, Nyce MR, Ohannesian JP, Marco CC, McKee LJ, Bauer TL, et al., 'Serum immunoreactive-leptin concentrations in normal-weight and obese humans', *N Engl J Med.* 1996 Feb 1; 334 (5): 292–5.

Cummings DE, Purnell JQ, Frayo RS, Schmidova K, Wisse BE, Weigle DS, 'A prandial rise in plasma ghrelin levels suggests a role in meal initiation in humans', *Diabetes* 2001 Aug; 50 (8): 1714–19.

Cummings DE, Weigle DS, Frayo RS, Breen PA, Ma MK, Dellinger EP, Purnell JQ, 'Plasma ghrelin levels after diet-induced weight loss or gastric bypass surgery', *N Engl J Med.* 2002 May 23; 346 (21): 1623–30.

De Silva A, Salem V, Long CJ, Makwana A, Newbould RD, Rabiner EA, Ghatei MA, Bloom SR, Matthews PM, Beaver JD, Dhillo WS, 'The gut hormones PYY 3-36 and GLP-1 7-36 amide reduce food intake and modulate brain activity in appetite centers in humans', *Cell Metab.* 2011 Nov 2; 14 (5): 700–6.

Denroche HC, Huynh FK, Kieffer TJ, 'The role of leptin in glucose homeostasis', *J Diabetes Investig.* 2012 Mar 28; 3 (2): 115–29.

Fothergill E, Guo J, Howard L, Kerns JC, Knuth ND, Brychta R, Chen KY, Skarulis MC, Walter M, Walter PJ, Hall KD, 'Persistent metabolic adaptation 6 years after "The Biggest Loser" competition', *Obesity (Silver Spring)* 2016 Aug; 24 (8): 1612–9.

Halaas JL, Gajiwala KS, Maffei M, Cohen SL, Chait BT, Rabinowitz D, Lallone RL, Burley SK, Friedman JM, 'Weight-reducing effects of the plasma protein encoded by the obese gene', *Science* 1995 Jul 28; 269 (5223): 543–6.

Hall KD, Ayuketah A, Brychta R, Cai H, Cassimatis T, Chen KY, Chung ST, Costa E, Courville A, Darcey V, Fletcher LA, Forde CG, Gharib AM, Guo J, Howard R, Joseph PV, McGehee S, Ouwerkerk R, Raisinger K, Rozga I, Stagliano M, Walter M, Walter PJ, Yang S, Zhou M, 'Ultra-Processed Diets Cause Excess Calorie Intake and Weight Gain: An Inpatient Randomized Controlled Trial of Ad Libitum Food Intake', *Cell Metab.* 2019 Jul 2; 30 (1): 67–77.e3.

Holst JJ, Madsbad S, Bojsen-Møller KN, Svane MS, Jørgensen NB, Dirksen C, Martinussen C, 'Mechanisms in bariatric surgery: Gut hormones, diabetes resolution, and weight loss', *Surg Obes Relat Dis.* 2018 May; 14 (5): 708–14.

Latner JD and Schwartz M, 'The effects of a high-carbohydrate, high-protein or balanced lunch upon later food intake and hunger ratings', *Appetite* 1999 Aug; 33 (1): 119–28.

Leibel RL, Rosenbaum M, Hirsch J, 'Changes in energy expenditure resulting from altered body weight', *N Engl J Med.* 1995 March 9; 332 (10): 621–8.

Lustig R, Sen S, Soberman J, Velasquez-Mieyer P, 'Obesity, leptin resistance, and the effects of insulin reduction', *Int J Obes.* 2004 Oct; 28 (10): 1344–8.

McConnon A, Horgan GW, Lawton C, Stubbs J, Shepherd R, Astrup A, Handjieva-Darlenska T, Kunešová M, Larsen TM, Lindroos AK, Martinez JA, Papadaki A, Pfeiffer AF, van Baak MA, Raats MM, 'Experience and acceptability of diets of varying protein content and glycemic index in an obese cohort: results from the Diogenes trial', *Eur J Clin Nutr.* 2013 Sep; 67 (9): 990–5.

Nakazato M, Murakami N, Date Y, Kojima M, Matsuo H, Kangawa K, Matsukura S, 'A role for ghrelin in the central regulation of feeding', *Nature* 2001 Jan 11; 409 (6817): 194–8.

Neel JV, 'Diabetes mellitus: a "thrifty" genotype rendered detrimental by "progress"?', *Am J Hum Genet.* 1962 Dec; 14 (4): 353–62.

Niswender KD, Schwartz MW, 'Insulin and leptin revisited: adiposity signals with overlapping physiological and intracellular signaling capabilities', *Front Neuroendocrinol.* 2003 Jan; 24 (1): 1–10.

Samra RA, 'Fats and Satiety'. In *Fat Detection: Taste, Texture, and Post Ingestive Effects*, ed. Montmayeur JP, le Coutre J (Boca Ranton (FL): CRC Press/Taylor & Francis, 2010).

Sumithran P, Prendergast LA, Delbridge E, Purcell K, Shulkes A, Kriketos A, Proietto J, 'Long-term persistence of hormonal adaptations to weight loss', *N Engl J Med.* 2011 Oct 27; 365 (17): 1597–1604.

Turton MD, O'Shea D, Gunn I, Beak SA, Edwards CM, Meeran K, Choi SJ, Taylor GM, Heath MM, Lambert PD, Wilding JP, Smith DM, Ghatei MA, Herbert J, Bloom SR, 'A role for glucagon-like peptide-1 in the central regulation of feeding', *Nature* 1996 Jan 4; 379 (6560): 69–72.

Wang J, Obici S, Morgan K, Barzilai N, Feng Z, Rossetti L, 'Overfeeding rapidly induces leptin and insulin resistance, *Diabetes* 2001 Dec; 50 (12): 2786–91.

Wren AM, Seal LJ, Cohen MA, Brynes AE, Frost GS, Murphy KG, Dhillo WS, Ghatei MA, Bloom SR, 'Ghrelin enhances appetite and increases food intake in humans,' *J Clin Endocrinol Metab.* 2001 Dec; 86 (12): 5992–5.

Zhang Y, Proenca R, Maffei M, Barone M, Leopold L, Friedman JM, 'Positional cloning of the mouse obese gene and its human homologue', *Nature* 1994 Dec 1; 372 (6505): 425–32.

Chapter 3: The Eating Window

Asher G and Sassone-Corsi P, 'Time for food: the intimate interplay between nutrition, metabolism, and the circadian clock', *Cell.* 2015 March 26; 161 (1): 84–92.

Chaix A, Zarrinpar A, Miu P, Panda S, 'Time-restricted feeding is a preventative and therapeutic intervention against diverse nutritional challenges', *Cell Metab.* 2014 Dec 2; 20 (6): 991–1005.

Dikic I and Elazar Z, 'Mechanism and medical implications of mammalian autophagy', *Nat Rev Mol Cell Biol.* 2018 Jun; 19 (6): 349–64.

Gallagher EJ and LeRoith D, 'Hyperinsulinaemia in cancer', *Nat Rev Cancer* 2020 Nov; 20 (11): 629–44.

Manoogian EN, Chow LS, Taub PR, Laferrère B, Panda S, 'Time-restricted eating for the prevention and management of metabolic diseases', *Endocr Rev.* 2021 Sep 22: bnab027. doi: 10.1210/endrev/bnab027. Epub ahead of print. PMID: 34550357.

Mattson MP, Moehl K, Ghena N, Schmaedick M, Cheng A, 'Intermittent metabolic switching, neuroplasticity and brain health', *Nat Rev Neurosci.* 2018 Feb; 19 (2): 63–80.

Nelson DL and Cox MM, 'Hormonal Regulation and Integration of Mammalian Metabolism (23.3) Hormonal Regulation of Fuel Metabolism.' In *Lehninger Principles of Biochemistry* seventh edition (New York: WH Freeman and Company, 2017), 930–939.

Pak HH, Haws SA, Green CL, Koller M, Lavarias MT, Richardson NE, Yang SE, Dumas SN, Sonsalla M, Bray L, Johnson M, Barnes S, Darley-Usmar V, Zhang J, Yen CE, Denu JM, Lamming DW, 'Fasting drives the metabolic, molecular and geroprotective effects of a calorie-restricted diet in mice', *Nat Metab.* 2021 Oct; 3 (10): 1327–41.

Sutton EF, Beyl R, Early KS, Cefalu WT, Ravussin E, Peterson CM, 'Early time-restricted feeding improves insulin sensitivity, blood pressure, and oxidative stress even without weight-loss in men with prediabetes', *Cell Metab.* 2018 Jun 5; 27 (6): 1212–21.

Um S, Frigerio F, Watanabe M, et al., 'Absence of S6K1 protects against age- and diet-induced obesity while enhancing insulin sensitivity', *Nature* 2004 Sep 9; 431 (7005): 200–205.

Vigneri R, Sciacca L, Vigneri P, 'Rethinking the Relationship between Insulin and Cancer', *Trends Endocrinol Metab.* 2020 Aug; 31 (8): 551–60.

Wilkinson MJ, Manoogian ENC, Zadourian A, Lo H, Fakhouri S, Shoghi A, Wang X, Fleischer JG, Navlakha S, Panda S, Taub PR, 'Ten-Hour Time-Restricted Eating Reduces Weight, Blood Pressure, and Atherogenic Lipids in Patients with Metabolic Syndrome', *Cell Metab.* 2020 Jan 7; 31 (1): 92–104.

Yang L, Li P, Fu S, Calay ES, Hotamisligil GS, 'Defective hepatic autophagy in obesity promotes ER stress and causes insulin resistance', *Cell Metab.* 2010 Jun 9; 11 (6): 467–78.

Youm YH, Nguyen KY, Grant RW, Goldberg EL, Bodogai M, Kim D, D'Agostino D, Planavsky N, Lupfer C, Kanneganti TD, Kang S, Horvath TL, Fahmy TM, Crawford PA, Biragyn A, Alnemri E, Dixit VD, 'The ketone metabolite β-hydroxybutyrate blocks NLRP3 inflammasome–mediated inflammatory disease', *Nat Med.* 2015 Mar; 21 (3): 263–9.

Zhu Y, Yan Y, Gius DR, Vassilopoulos A, 'Metabolic regulation of Sirtuins upon fasting and the implication for cancer', *Curr Opin Oncol.* 2013; 25 (6): 630–6.

Chapter 4: Gut bacteria

Breton J, Tennoune N, Lucas N, Francois M, Legrand R, Jacquemot J, Goichon A, Guérin C, Peltier J, Pestel-Caron M,

Chan P, Vaudry D, do Rego JC, Liénard F, Pénicaud L, Fioramonti X, Ebenezer IS, Hökfelt T, Déchelotte P, Fetissov SO, 'Gut Commensal E. coli Proteins Activate Host Satiety Pathways following Nutrient-Induced Bacterial Growth', *Cell Metab.* 2016 Feb 9; 23 (2): 324–34.

Cammarota G, Ianiro G, Kelly CR, Mullish BH, Allegretti JR, Kassam Z, Putignani L, Fischer M, Keller JJ, Costello SP, Sokol H, Kump P, Satokari R, Kahn SA, Kao D, Arkkila P, Kuijper EJ, Vehreschild MJG, Pintus C, Lopetuso L, Masucci L, Scaldaferri F, Terveer EM, Nieuwdorp M, López-Sanromán A, Kupcinskas J, Hart A, Tilg H, Gasbarrini A, 'International consensus conference on stool banking for faecal microbiota transplantation in clinical practice', *Gut* 2019 Dec; 68 (12): 2111–21.

Chassaing B, Koren O, Goodrich JK, Poole AC, Srinivasan S, Ley RE, Gewirtz AT, 'Dietary emulsifiers impact the mouse gut microbiota promoting colitis and metabolic syndrome', *Nature* 2015 Mar 5; 519 (7541): 92–6.

David LA, Maurice CF, Carmody RN, Gootenberg DB, Button JE, Wolfe BE, Ling AV, Devlin AS, Varma Y, Fischbach MA, Biddinger SB, Dutton RJ, Turnbaugh PJ, 'Diet rapidly and reproducibly alters the human gut microbiome', *Nature* 2014 Jan 23; 505 (7484): 559–63.

Dominique M, Breton J, Guérin C, Bole-Feysot C, Lambert G, Déchelotte P, Fetissov S, 'Effects of macronutrients on the in vitro production of ClpB, a bacterial mimetic protein of α-MSH and its possible role in satiety signaling', *Nutrients* 2019 Sep 5; 11 (9): 2115.

Fetissov S, 'Role of the gut microbiota in host appetite control: bacterial growth to animal feeding behaviour', *Nat Rev Endocrinol.* 2017 Jan; 13 (1): 11–25.

Ley RE, Bäckhed F, Turnbaugh P, Lozupone CA, Knight RD, Gordon JI 'Obesity alters gut microbial ecology', *Proc Natl Acad Sci USA* 2005 Aug 2; 102 (31): 11070–5.

REFERENCES

Ley RE, Turnbaugh PJ, Klein S, Gordon JI, 'Microbial ecology: human gut microbes associated with obesity', *Nature* 2006 Dec 21; 444 (7122): 1022–3.

Li Z, Yi CX, Katiraei S, Kooijman S, Zhou E, Chung CK, Gao Y, van den Heuvel JK, Meijer OC, Berbée JFP, Heijink M, Giera M, Willems van Dijk K, Groen AK, Rensen PCN, Wang Y, 'Butyrate reduces appetite and activates brown adipose tissue via the gut–brain neural circuit', *Gut* 2018 Jul; 67 (7): 1269–79.

Martel J, Ojcius DM, Chang CJ, Lin CS, Lu CC, Ko YF, Tseng SF, Lai HC, Young JD, 'Anti-obesogenic and antidiabetic effects of plants and mushrooms,' *Nat Rev Endocrinol.* 2017 Mar; 13 (3): 149–60.

Mazloom K, Siddiqi I, Covasa M, 'Probiotics: How Effective Are They in the Fight against Obesity?' *Nutrients* 2019 Jan 24; 11 (2): 258.

Moeller AH, Caro-Quintero A, Mjungu D, Georgiev AV, Lonsdorf EV, Muller MN, Pusey AE, Peeters M, Hahn BH, Ochman H, 'Cospeciation of gut microbiota with hominids', *Science* 2016 Jul 22; 353 (6297): 380–2.

Parks BW, Nam E, Org E, Kostem E, Norheim F, Hui ST, Pan C, Civelek M, Rau CD, Bennett BJ, Mehrabian M, Ursell LK, He A, Castellani LW, Zinker B, Kirby M, Drake TA, Drevon CA, Knight R, Gargalovic P, Kirchgessner T, Eskin E, Lusis AJ, 'Genetic control of obesity and gut microbiota composition in response to high-fat, high-sucrose diet in mice', *Cell Metab.* 2013 Jan 8; 17 (1): 141–52.

Schwiertz A, Taras D, Schäfer K, Beijer S, Bos NA, Donus C, Hardt PD, 'Microbiota and SCFA in lean and overweight healthy subjects', *Obesity (Silver Spring)* 2010 Jan; 18 (1): 190–5.

Scientific Advisory Committee on Nutrition, 'Carbohydrates and health'. Published 2015. London: The Stationery Office. Available at: https://assets.publishing.service.gov.uk/government/uploads/system/uploads/attachment_data/file/445503/SACN_Carbohydrates_and_Health.pdf

Silva YP, Bernardi A and Frozza RL, 'The Role of Short-Chain Fatty Acids From Gut Microbiota in Gut–Brain Communication', *Front. Endocrinol.* (Lausanne) 2020 Jan 31; 11: 25.

Sonnenburg ED, Smits SA, Tikhonov M, Higginbottom SK, Wingreen NS, Sonnenburg JL, 'Diet-induced extinctions in the gut microbiota compound over generations', *Nature* 2016 Jan 14; 529 (7585): 212–5.

Suez J, Korem T, Zeevi D, Zilberman-Schapira G, Thaiss CA, Maza O, Israeli D, Zmora N, Gilad S, Weinberger A, Kuperman Y, Harmelin A, Kolodkin-Gal I, Shapiro H, Halpern Z, Segal E, Elinav E, 'Artificial sweeteners induce glucose intolerance by altering the gut microbiota', *Nature* 2014 Oct 9; 514 (7521): 181–6.

Turnbaugh PJ, Ley RE, Mahowald MA, Magrini V, Mardis ER, Gordon JI, 'An obesity-associated gut microbiome with increased capacity for energy harvest', *Nature* 2006 Dec 21; 444 (7122): 1027–31.

Vijay-Kumar M, Aitken JD, Carvalho FA, Cullender TC, Mwangi S, Srinivasan S, Sitaraman SV, Knight R, Ley RE, Gewirtz AT, 'Metabolic syndrome and altered gut microbiota in mice lacking Toll-like receptor 5', *Science* 2010 Apr 9; 328 (5975): 228–31.

Wong JM, de Souza R, Kendall CW, Emam A, Jenkins DJ, 'Colonic Health: Fermentation and Short Chain Fatty Acids', *Journal of Clinical Gastroenterology*, 2006; 40 (3): 235–43.

Wu GD, Chen J, Hoffmann C, Bittinger K, Chen YY, Keilbaugh SA, Bewtra M, Knights D, Walters WA, Knight R, Sinha R, Gilroy E, Gupta K, Baldassano R, Nessel L, Li H, Bushman FD, Lewis JD, 'Linking long-term dietary patterns with gut microbial enterotypes', *Science* 2011 Oct 7; 334 (6052): 105–8.

Chapter 5: Movement

Althoff T, Sosič R, Hicks JL, King AC, Delp SL, Leskovec J, 'Large-scale physical activity data reveal worldwide activity inequality', *Nature* 2017 Jul 20; 547 (7663): 336–9.

Aragno M and Mastrocola R, 'Dietary Sugars and Endogenous Formation of Advanced Glycation Endproducts: Emerging Mechanisms of Disease', *Nutrients* 2017; 9 (4): 385.

Brownie AC and Kernohan JC, 'Integration of metabolism'. In *Master Medicine: Medical Biochemistry: A core text with self-assessment* second edition (Churchill Livingstone, 2005), 145–162.

Chan JSY, Liu G, Liang D, Deng K, Wu J, Yan JH, 'Special issue – therapeutic benefits of physical activity for mood: a systematic review on the effects of exercise intensity, duration, and modality', *J Psychol.* 2019; 153 (1): 102–25.

Chia CW, Egan JM, Ferrucci L, 'Age-Related Changes in Glucose Metabolism, Hyperglycemia, and Cardiovascular Risk', *Circ Res.* 2018 Sep 14; 123 (7): 886–904.

Czech M, 'Insulin action and resistance in obesity and type 2 diabetes', *Nat Med.* 2017 Jul 11: 23 (7): 804–14.

Dolezal BA, Neufeld EV, Boland DM, Martin JL, Cooper CB, 'Interrelationship between Sleep and Exercise: A Systematic Review', *Adv Prev Med.* 2017; 2017: 1364387.

Eckel RH, Grundy SM, Zimmet PZ, 'The metabolic syndrome', *Lancet* 2005 Apr 16–22; 365 (9468): 1415–28.

Escobar-Morreale HF, 'Polycystic ovary syndrome: definition, aetiology, diagnosis and treatment', *Nat Rev Endocrinol.* 2018 May; 14 (5): 270–84.

Garfield V, Farmaki AE, Eastwood SV, Mathur R, Rentsch CT, Bhaskaran K, Smeeth L, Chaturvedi N, 'HbA1c and brain health across the entire glycaemic spectrum', *Diabetes Obes Metab.* 2021 May; 23 (5): 1140–9.

Goh SY and Cooper ME, 'Clinical review: The role of advanced glycation end products in progression and complications of diabetes', *J Clin Endocrinol Metab.* 2008 Apr; 93 (4): 1143–52.

Huang Y, Cai X, Mai W, Li M, Hu Y, 'Association between prediabetes and risk of cardiovascular disease and all cause mortality: systematic review and meta-analysis', *BMJ* 2016 Nov 23; 355: i5953.

Kahn S, Hull R, Utzschneider K, 'Mechanisms linking obesity to insulin resistance and type 2 diabetes', *Nature* 2006 Dec 14; 444 (7121): 840–6.

Levine JA, Vander Weg MW, Hill JO, Klesges RC, 'Non-exercise activity thermogenesis. The crouching tiger hidden dragon of societal weight gain', *Arteriosclerosis, Thrombosis, and Vascular Biology* 2006 Apr; 26 (4): 729–36.

Lim B, 'Exercising for a stronger heart'. In *Keeping your heart healthy.* (London: Penguin Life, 2021).

Naci H and Ioannidis JP, 'Comparative effectiveness of exercise and drug interventions on mortality outcomes: metaepidemiological study', *BMJ* 2013 Oct 1; 347: f5577.

Vina J, Sanchis-Gomar F, Martinez-Bello V, Gomez-Cabrera MC, 'Exercise acts as a drug; the pharmacological benefits of exercise', *Br J Pharmacol.* 2012 Sep; 167 (1): 1–12.

Chapter 6: Sleep

Benedict C, Brooks SJ, O'Daly OG, Almèn MS, Morell A, Åberg K, Gingnell M, Schultes B, Hallschmid M, Broman JE, Larsson EM, Schiöth HB, 'Acute sleep deprivation enhances the brain's response to hedonic food stimuli: an fMRI study', *J Clin Endocrinol Metab.* 2012 Mar; 97 (3): E443–7.

Brondel L, Romer MA, Nougues PM, Touyarou P, Davenne D, 'Acute partial sleep deprivation increases food intake in healthy men', *Am J Clin Nutr.* 2010 Jun; 91 (6): 1550–9.

Donga E, van Dijk M, van Dijk JG, Biermasz NR, Lammers GJ, van Kralingen KW, Corssmit EP, Romijn JA, 'A single night of partial sleep deprivation induces insulin resistance in multiple metabolic pathways in healthy subjects', *J Clin Endocrinol Metab.* 2010 Jun; 95 (6): 2963–8.

Foster RG, 'Sleep, circadian rhythms and health', *Interface Focus* 2020 Jun 6; 10 (3): 20190098.

Fultz NE, Bonmassar G, Setsompop K, Stickgold RA, Rosen BR, Polimeni JR, Lewis LD, 'Coupled electrophysiological, hemodynamic, and cerebrospinal fluid oscillations in human sleep', *Science* 2019 Nov 1; 366 (6465): 628–31.

Hastings MH, Maywood ES, Brancaccio M, 'Generation of circadian rhythms in the suprachiasmatic nucleus', *Nat Rev Neurosci.* 2018 Aug; 19 (8): 453–69.

Hastings MH, Reddy AB, Maywood ES, 'A clockwork web: Circadian timing in brain and periphery, in health and disease', *Nat Rev Neurosci.* 2003 Aug; 4 (8): 649–61.

Kredlow MA, Capozzoli MC, Hearon BA, Calkins AW, Otto MW, 'The effects of physical activity on sleep: a meta-analytic review', *J Behav Med.* 2015 Jun; 38 (3): 427–49.

Meerlo P, Sgoifo A, Suchecki D, 'Restricted and disrupted sleep: effects on autonomic function, neuroendocrine stress systems and stress responsivity', *Sleep Med Rev.* 2008 Jun; 12 (3): 197–210.

Michel S, Meijer JH, 'From clock to functional pacemaker', *Eur J Neurosci.* 2020 Jan; 51(1): 482–93.

Nehlig A, 'Interindividual Differences in Caffeine Metabolism and Factors Driving Caffeine Consumption', *Pharmacol Rev.* 2018 Apr; 70 (2): 384–411.

Nikbakhtian S, Reed AB, Obika BD, Morelli D, Cunningham AC, Aral M, Plans D, 'Accelerometer-derived sleep onset timing and cardiovascular disease incidence: a UK Biobank cohort study', *European Heart Journal – Digital Health.* Published 2021 Dec; 2 (4): 658–66

Okamoto-Mizuno K, Mizuno K, 'Effects of thermal environment on sleep and circadian rhythm', *J Physiol Anthropol.* 2012 May 31; 31 (1): 14.

Scheer FA, Hilton MF, Mantzoros CS, Shea SA, 'Adverse metabolic and cardiovascular consequences of circadian misalignment', *PNAS.* 2009 Mar 17; 106 (11): 4453–8.

Spiegel K, Knutson K, Leproult R, Tasali E, Van Cauter E 'Sleep loss: a novel risk factor for insulin resistance and Type 2 diabetes', *J Appl Physiol.* (1985). 2005 Nov; 99 (5): 2008–19.

Spiegel K, Leproult R, Van Cauter E, 'Impact of sleep debt on metabolic and endocrine function', *Lancet* 1999 Oct 23; 354 (9188): 1435–9.

Taheri S, Lin L, Austin D, Young T, Mignot E, 'Short sleep duration is associated with reduced leptin, elevated ghrelin, and increased body mass index', *PLoS Med.* 2004 Dec; 1 (3): e62.

Tosini G, Ferguson I, Tsubota K, 'Effects of blue light on the circadian system and eye physiology', *Mol Vis.* 2016 Jan 24; 22: 61–72.

Chapter 7: Genes

Bouchard C, Tremblay A, Després JP, Nadeau A, Lupien PJ, Thériault G, Dussault J, Moorjani S, Pinault S, Fournier G, 'The response to long-term overfeeding in identical twins', *N Engl J Med.* 1990 May 24; 322 (21): 1477–82.

Cecil JE, Tavendale R, Watt P, Hetherington MM, Palmer CN, 'An obesity-associated FTO gene variant and increased energy intake in children', *N Engl J Med.* 2008 Dec 11; 359 (24): 2558–66.

Cribb J, Johnson P, Joyce R, Oldfield Z, 'Jubilees compared: incomes, spending and work in the late 1970s and early 2010s', IFS Briefing Note BN128. Institute for Fiscal Studies. 2012. Available at: https://ifs.org.uk/bns/bn128.pdf

Department for Environment, Food and Rural Affairs (DEFRA) National Statistics – 'Food Statistics in your pocket: Prices and expenditure'. Updated 30 November 2020. Available at: https://www.gov.uk/government/statistics/food-statistics-pocketbook/food-statistics-in-your-pocket-prices-and-expenditure

Farooqi S and O'Rahilly S, 'Genetics of obesity in humans', *Endocr Rev.* 2006 Dec; 27 (7): 710–18.

Frayling TM, Timpson NJ, Weedon MN, Zeggini E, Freathy RM, Lindgren CM, Perry JR, Elliott KS, Lango H, Rayner NW, Shields B, Harries LW, Barrett JC, Ellard S, Groves CJ, Knight B, Patch AM, Ness AR, Ebrahim S, Lawlor DA, Ring SM, Ben-Shlomo Y, Jarvelin MR, Sovio U, Bennett AJ, Melzer D, Ferrucci L, Loos RJ, Barroso I, Wareham NJ, Karpe F, Owen KR, Cardon LR, Walker M, Hitman GA, Palmer CN, Doney AS, Morris AD, Smith GD, Hattersley AT, McCarthy MI, 'A common variant in the FTO gene is associated with body mass index and predisposes to childhood and adult obesity', *Science* 2007 May 11; 316 (5826): 889–94.

Llewellyn CH, Trzaskowski M, van Jaarsveld CHM, Plomin R, Wardle J, 'Satiety Mechanisms in Genetic Risk of Obesity', *JAMA Pediatr.* 2014 Apr; 168 (4): 338–44.

Melhorn SJ, Askren MK, Chung WK, Kratz M, Bosch TA, Tyagi V, Webb MF, De Leon MRB, Grabowski TJ, Leibel RL, Schur EA,

'FTO genotype impacts food intake and corticolimbic activation', *Am J Clin Nutr.* 2018 Feb 1; 107 (2): 145–54.

Murray S, Tulloch A, Gold MS, Avena NM, 'Hormonal and neural mechanisms of food reward, eating behaviour and obesity', *Nat Rev Endocrinol.* 2014 Sep; 10 (9): 540–52.

Neel JV, 'Diabetes mellitus: a "thrifty" genotype rendered detrimental by "progress"?', *Am J Hum Genet.* 1962 Dec; 14 (4): 353–62.

NHS Digital, Health Survey for England, 2019: 'Overweight and obesity in adults and children'. Published 2020. Available at: https://digital.nhs.uk/data-andinformation/publications/statistical/health-survey-for-england

Rosenbaum S, Skinner RK, Knight IB, Garrow JS, 'A survey of heights and weights of adults in Great Britain, 1980', *Ann Hum Biol.* 1985 Mar–Apr; 12 (2): 115–27.

Stice E, Spoor S, Bohon C, Small DM, 'Relation between obesity and blunted striatal response to food is moderated by TaqIA A1 allele', *Science* 2008 Oct 17; 322 (5900): 449–52.

Stunkard AJ, Harris JR, Pedersen NL, McClearn GE, 'The body-mass index of twins who have been reared apart', *N Engl J Med.* 1990 May 24; 322 (21): 1483–7.

Tung YCL, Yeo GSH, O'Rahilly S, Coll AP, 'Obesity and FTO: Changing Focus at a Complex Locus', *Cell Metab.* 2014 Nov 4; 20 (5): 710–18.

Wang GJ, Volkow ND, Logan J, Pappas NR, Wong CT, Zhu W, Netusil N, Fowler JS, 'Brain dopamine and obesity', *Lancet* 2001 Feb 3; 357 (9253): 354–7.

Chapter 8: The food industry

American Psychiatric Association, 'Substance-related and Addictive Disorders'. In *Diagnostic and Statistical Manual of Mental Disorders* fifth edition (Arlington, VA: American Psychiatric Association, 2013), 481–589.

Chang K, Khandpur N, Neri D, Touvier M, Huybrechts I, Millett C, Vamos EP, 'Association Between Childhood Consumption of Ultraprocessed Food and Adiposity Trajectories in the Avon Longitudinal Study of Parents and Children Birth Cohort', *JAMA Pediatr.* 2021 Sep 1; 175 (9): e211573.

Cordova R, Kliemann N, Huybrechts I, Rauber F, Vamos EP, Levy RB, Wagner KH, Viallon V, Casagrande C, Nicolas G, Dahm CC, Zhang J, Halkjær J, Tjønneland A, Boutron-Ruault MC, Mancini FR, Laouali N, Katzke V, Srour B, Jannasch F, Schulze MB, Masala G, Grioni S, Panico S, van der Schouw YT, Derksen JWG, Rylander C, Skeie G, Jakszyn P, Rodriguez-Barranco M, Huerta JM, Barricarte A, Brunkwall L, Ramne S, Bodén S, Perez-Cornago A, Heath AK, Vineis P, Weiderpass E, Monteiro CA, Gunter MJ, Millett C, Freisling H, 'Consumption of ultra-processed foods associated with weight gain and obesity in adults: A multi-national cohort study', *Clin Nutr.* 2021 Sep; 40 (9): 5079–88.

Fiolet T, Srour B, Sellem L, Kesse-Guyot E, Allès B, Méjean C, Deschasaux M, Fassier P, Latino-Martel P, Beslay M, Hercberg S, Lavalette C, Monteiro CA, Julia C, Touvier M, 'Consumption of ultra-processed foods and cancer risk: results from NutriNet-Santé prospective cohort', *BMJ* 2018 Feb 14; 360: k322.

Hall KD, Ayuketah A, Brychta R, Cai H, Cassimatis T, Chen KY, Chung ST, Costa E, Courville A, Darcey V, Fletcher LA, Forde CG, Gharib AM, Guo J, Howard R, Joseph PV, McGehee S, Ouwerkerk R, Raisinger K, Rozga I, Stagliano M, Walter M, Walter PJ, Yang S, Zhou M, 'Ultra-Processed Diets Cause Excess Calorie

Intake and Weight Gain: An Inpatient Randomized Controlled Trial of Ad Libitum Food Intake', *Cell Metab.* 2019 Jul 2; 30 (1): 67–77.e3.

Johnson PM and Kenny PJ, 'Dopamine D2 receptors in addiction-like reward dysfunction and compulsive eating in obese rats', *Nat Neurosci.* 2010 May; 13 (5): 635–41.

Lenoir M, Serre F, Cantin L, Ahmed SH, 'Intense sweetness surpasses cocaine reward', *PLoS One* 2007 Aug 1; 2 (8): e698.

McCann D, Barrett A, Cooper A, Crumpler D, Dalen L, Grimshaw K, Kitchin E, Lok K, Porteous L, Prince E, Sonuga-Barke E, Warner JO, Stevenson J, 'Food additives and hyperactive behaviour in 3-year-old and 8/9-year-old children in the community: a randomised, double-blinded, placebo-controlled trial', *Lancet* 2007 Nov 3; 370 (9598): 1560–7.

Monteiro CA, Cannon G, Lawrence M, Costa Louzada ML, Pereira Machado P, 'Ultra-processed foods, diet quality, and health using the NOVA classification system', Food and Agriculture Organization of the United Nations (FAO). 2019. Available at: http://www.fao.org/3/ca5644en/ca5644en.pdf

Monteiro CA, Cannon G, Moubarac JC, Levy RB, Louzada MLC, Jaime PC, 'The UN Decade of Nutrition, the NOVA food classification and the trouble with ultra-processing', *Public Health Nutr.* 2018 Jan; 21 (1): 5–17.

Moss, M, *Salt, Sugar, Fat: How the Food Giants Hooked Us* (WH Allen, 2014).

Rauber F, Louzada MLDC, Martinez Steele E, Rezende LFM, Millett C, Monteiro CA, Levy RB, 'Ultra-processed foods and excessive free sugar intake in the UK: a nationally representative cross-sectional study', *BMJ Open* 2019 Oct 28; 9 (10): e027546.

Rauber F, Steele EM, Louzada MLDC, Millett C, Monteiro CA, Levy RB, 'Ultra-processed food consumption and indicators of obesity in the United Kingdom population (2008–2016)', *PLoS One* 2020 May 1; 15 (5): e0232676.

Stuckler D and Nestle M, 'Big food, food systems, and global health', *PLoS Med.* 2012; 9 (6): e1001242.

Chapter 9: History lessons

Buettner D and Skemp S, 'Blue Zones: Lessons From the World's Longest Lived', *Am J Lifestyle Med.* 2016 Jul 7; 10 (5): 318–21.

Delamothe T, 'Founding principles', *BMJ.* 2008 May 31; 336 (7655): 1216–8.

Hex N, Bartlett C, Wright D, Taylor M, Varley D, 'Estimating the current and future costs of Type 1 and Type 2 diabetes in the UK, including direct health costs and indirect societal and productivity costs', *Diabet Med.* 2012 Jul; 29 (7): 855–62.

Himsworth HP, 'The syndrome of diabetes mellitus and its causes', *Lancet* 1949 Mar 19; 1 (6551): 465–73.

Holland WW and Stewart S, 'Public Health: The vision and the challenge', The Rock Carling Fellowship 1997. Published by The Nuffield Trust. 1998. Available at: https://www.nuffieldtrust.org.uk/files/2017-01/public-health-vision-challenge-web-final.pdf

Ministry of Food, 'This Week's Food Facts No.1: Grow fit not fat on your war diet. Make full use of the fruit and vegetables in season. Cut out 'extras', cut out waste; don't eat more than you need.' 1940.

Ministry of Health, 'A National Health Service'. Presented by the Minister of Health and the Secretary of State for Scotland to Parliament by Command of His Majesty February. London.

Published by His Majesty's Stationery Office (HMSO). London 1944.

Public Health England, 'A Century of Public Health Marketing. Enduring public health challenges and revolutions in communication'. 2017. Available at: https://publichealthengland. exposure.co/100-years-of-public-health-marketing

Rivett, G, *The history of the NHS*. Available at: https://www. nuffieldtrust.org.uk/health-and-social-care-explained/the-history-of-the-nhs

Whicher CA, O'Neill S, Holt RIG, 'Diabetes in the UK: 2019', *Diabet Med.* 2020 Feb; 37 (2): 242–7.

Young FG, Richardson KC, et al., 'Discussion on the cause of diabetes', *Proc R Soc Med.* 1949 May; 42 (5): 321–30.

Chapter 10: Language

Bannister R, *The Four-Minute Mile* (Lyons Press, 2018).

Draganski B, Gaser C, Busch V, Schuierer G, Bogdahn U, May A, 'Neuroplasticity: changes in grey matter induced by training', *Nature* 2004 Jan 22; 427 (6972): 311–2.

ESPN Films and Netflix, *The Last Dance*, directed by Jason Hehir. Episode X. 2020. Available at: www.netflix.com

Feldman S, Conforti N, Weidenfeld J, 'Limbic pathways and hypothalamic neurotransmitters mediating adrenocortical responses to neural stimuli', *Neurosci Biobehav Rev.* 1995 Summer; 19 (2): 235–40.

Fowler JH and Christakis NA, 'Dynamic spread of happiness in a large social network: longitudinal analysis over 20 years in the Framingham Heart Study', *BMJ* 2008 Dec 4; 337: a2338.

Hatfield E, Cacioppo JT, Rapson RL, 'Emotional Contagion', *Current Directions in Psychological Science* 1993; 2 (3): 96–100.

Kandel ER, Schwartz JH, Jessell TM, Siegelbaum SA, Hudspeth AJ, eds. 'The Organization of Cognition'. In *Principles of Neural Science* fifth edition (McGraw-Hill, 2012), 392–411.

Li Y, Lopez-Huerta VG, Adiconis X, Levandowski K, Choi S, Simmons SK, Arias-Garcia MA, Guo B, Yao AY, Blosser TR, Wimmer RD, Aida T, Atamian A, Naik T, Sun X, Bi D, Malhotra D, Hession CC, Shema R, Gomes M, Li T, Hwang E, Krol A, Kowalczyk M, Peça J, Pan G, Halassa MM, Levin JZ, Fu Z, Feng G, 'Distinct subnetworks of the thalamic reticular nucleus', *Nature* 2020 Jul; 583 (7818): 819–824.

Longe O, Maratos FA, Gilbert P, Evans G, Volker F, Rockliff H, Rippon G, 'Having a word with yourself: neural correlates of self-criticism and self-reassurance', *Neuroimage* 2010 Jan 15; 49 (2): 1849–56.

Meyer-Lindenberg A, Domes G, Kirsch P, Heinrichs M, 'Oxytocin and vasopressin in the human brain: social neuropeptides for translational medicine', *Nat Rev Neurosci.* 2011 Aug 19; 12 (9): 524–38.

Nakajima M, Schmitt LI, Halassa MM, 'Prefrontal Cortex Regulates Sensory Filtering through a Basal Ganglia-to-Thalamus Pathway', *Neuron* 2019 Aug 7; 103 (3): 445-458.e10.

Neck CP and Manz CC, 'Thought self-leadership: The influence of self-talk and mental imagery on performance', *Journal of Organizational Behavior* 1992 Dec; 13: 681–99.

Posner MI, Rueda MR, Kanske P, 'Probing the mechanisms of attention'. In *Handbook of Psychophysiology*, ed. Cacioppo JT, Tassinary LG, Berntson GG (Cambridge: Cambridge University Press, 2007), 410–32.

Wimmer RD, Schmitt LI, Davidson TJ, Nakajima M, Deisseroth K, Halassa MM, 'Thalamic control of sensory selection in divided attention', *Nature* 2015; 526: 705–709.

Yin H and Knowlton B, 'The role of the basal ganglia in habit formation', *Nat Rev Neurosci.* 2006 Jun; 7 (6): 464–76.

Zhu Y, Nachtrab G, Keyes PC, Allen WE, Luo L, Chen X, 'Dynamic salience processing in paraventricular thalamus gates associative learning', *Science* 2018 Oct 26; 362 (6413): 423–429.

Chapter 11: Goals

Gollwitzer PM, 'Implementation intentions: strong effects of simple plans', *American Psychologist* 1999 Jul; 54 (7): 493–503.

Hameed S, Salem V, Alessimii H, Scholtz S, Dar O, Miras AD, Meeran K, Bloom SR, Ahmed AR, Purkayastha S, Chahal H, Tan T, 'Imperial Satiety Protocol: A new non-surgical weight-loss programme, delivered in a health care setting, produces improved clinical outcomes for people with obesity', *Diabetes Obes Metab.* 2021 Jan; 23 (1): 270–5.

Johnson, M, *Gold Rush: What makes an Olympic champion?* (Harper Sport, 2012).

Locke EA and Latham GP, 'Building a practically useful theory of goal setting and task motivation. A 35-year odyssey', *Am Psychol.* 2002 Sep; 57 (9): 705–17.

Pearson J, 'The human imagination: the cognitive neuroscience of visual mental imagery', *Nat Rev Neurosci.* 2019 Oct; 20 (10): 624–34.

Solbrig L, Whalley B, Kavanagh DJ, May J, Parkin T, Jones R, Andrade J, 'Functional imagery training versus motivational interviewing for weight loss: a randomised controlled trial of brief individual interventions for overweight and obesity', *Int J Obes (Lond)*. 2019 Apr; 43 (4): 883–94.

Thaler RH and Sunstein CR, *Nudge: Improving Decisions About Health, Wealth, and Happiness* (New Haven, CT: Yale University Press, 2008).

Chapter 12: Brain gains

Bruze G, Holmin TE, Peltonen M, Ottosson J, Sjöholm K, Näslund I, Neovius M, Carlsson LMS, Svensson PA, 'Associations of Bariatric Surgery with Changes in Interpersonal Relationship Status: Results From 2 Swedish Cohort Studies', *JAMA Surg*. 2018 Jul 1; 153 (7): 654–61.

Catani M, Dell'acqua F, Thiebaut de Schotten M, 'A revised limbic system model for memory, emotion and behaviour', *Neurosci Biobehav Rev*. 2013 Sep; 37 (8): 1724–37.

Diamond A, 'Executive functions', *Annu Rev Psychol*. 2013; 64: 135–68.

Felitti VJ, Anda RF, Nordenberg D, Williamson DF, Spitz AM, Edwards V, Koss MP, Marks JS, 'Relationship of childhood abuse and household dysfunction to many of the leading causes of death in adults. The Adverse Childhood Experiences (ACE) Study', *Am J Prev Med*. 1998 May; 14 (4): 245–58.

Felitti VJ, Jakstis K, Pepper V, Ray A, 'Obesity: problem, solution, or both?' *Perm J*. 2010 Spring; 14 (1): 24–30.

Fishbain DA, Rosomoff HL, Cutler RB, Rosomoff RS, 'Secondary gain concept: a review of the scientific evidence', *Clin J Pain*. 1995 Mar; 11 (1): 6–21.

Goldin PR, McRae K, Ramel W, Gross JJ, 'The neural bases of emotion regulation: reappraisal and suppression of negative emotion', *Biol Psychiatry*. 2008 Mar 15; 63 (6): 577–86.

Kandel ER, Schwartz JH, Jessell TM, Siegelbaum SA, Hudspeth AJ, eds. 'Emotions and Feelings'. In *Principles of Neural Science* fifth edition (McGraw-Hill, 2012), 1079–94.

Neill JR, Marshall JR, Yale CE, 'Marital changes after intestinal bypass surgery', *JAMA*. 1978 Aug 4; 240 (5): 447–58.

Ohman A, 'The role of the amygdala in human fear: automatic detection of threat', *Psychoneuroendocrinology* 2005 Nov; 30 (10): 953–8.

Salem V, Demetriou L, Behary P, Alexiadou K, Scholtz S, Tharakan G, Miras AD, Purkayastha S, Ahmed AR, Bloom SR, Wall MB, Dhillo WS, Tan TM, 'Weight Loss by Low-Calorie Diet Versus Gastric Bypass Surgery in People with Diabetes Results in Divergent Brain Activation Patterns: A Functional MRI Study', *Diabetes Care* 2021 Aug; 44 (8): 1842–51.

Williamson DF, Thompson TJ, Anda RF, Dietz WH, Felitti V, 'Body weight and obesity in adults and self-reported abuse in childhood', *Int J Obes Relat Metab Disord.* 2002 Aug; 26 (8): 1075–82.

Chapter 13: Feelings

Blum K, Braverman ER, Holder JM, Lubar JF, Monastra VJ, Miller D, Lubar JO, Chen TJ, Comings DE, 'Reward deficiency syndrome: a biogenetic model for the diagnosis and treatment of impulsive, addictive, and compulsive behaviors', *Journal of Psychoactive Drugs* 2000 Nov; 32 (Suppl i–iv): 1–112.

Firth J, Gangwisch JE, Borisini A, Wootton RE, Mayer EA, 'Food and mood: how do diet and nutrition affect mental wellbeing?' *BMJ* 2020 Jun 29; 369: m2382.

Fung TC, Vuong HE, Luna CDG, Pronovost GN, Aleksandrova AA, Riley NG, Vavilina A, McGinn J, Rendon T, Forrest LR, Hsiao EY, 'Intestinal serotonin and fluoxetine exposure modulate bacterial colonization in the gut', *Nat Microbiol.* 2019 Dec; 4 (12): 2064–73.

Gupta A, Osadchiy V, Mayer EA, 'Brain–gut–microbiome interactions in obesity and food addiction', *Nat Rev Gastroenterol Hepatol.* 2020 Nov; 17 (11): 655–72.

Hameed S, Salem V, Alessimii H, Scholtz S, Dar O, Miras AD, Meeran K, Bloom SR, Ahmed AR, Purkayastha S, Chahal H, Tan T, 'Imperial Satiety Protocol: A new non-surgical weight-loss programme, delivered in a health care setting, produces improved clinical outcomes for people with obesity', *Diabetes Obes Metab.* 2021 Jan; 23 (1): 270–5.

Jastreboff AM, Sinha R, Lacadie C, Small DM, Sherwin RS, Potenza MN, 'Neural correlates of stress- and food cue-induced food craving in obesity: association with insulin levels', *Diabetes Care* 2013 Feb; 36 (2): 394–402.

Mayer EA, 'Gut feelings: the emerging biology of gut–brain communication', *Nat Rev Neurosci.* 2011 Jul 13; 12 (8): 453–66.

Shin AC, Zheng H, Berthoud HR, 'An expanded view of energy homeostasis: neural integration of metabolic, cognitive, and emotional drives to eat', *Physiology & Behavior* 2009 Jul 14; 97 (5): 572–80.

Steinsbekk S, Barker ED, Llewellyn C, Fildes A, Wichstrøm L, 'Emotional Feeding and Emotional Eating: Reciprocal Processes and the Influence of Negative Affectivity', *Child Dev.* 2018 Jul; 89 (4): 1234–46.

Stice E, Spoor S, Bohon C, Small DM, 'Relation between obesity and blunted striatal response to food is moderated by TaqIA A1 allele', *Science* 2008 Oct 17; 322 (5900): 449–52.

Volkow ND, Wang GJ, Maynard L, Jayne M, Fowler JS, Zhu W, Logan J, Gatley SJ, Ding YS, Wong C, Pappas N, 'Brain dopamine is associated with eating behavior in humans', *International Journal of Eating Disorders* 2003 Mar; 33 (2): 136–42.

Wang GJ, Volkow ND, Logan J, Pappas NR, Wong C, Zhu W, Netsuil N, Fowler NS, 'Brain dopamine and obesity', *Lancet* 2001 Feb 3; 357 (9253): 354–7.

Wang YB, de Lartigue G, Page AJ, 'Dissecting the Role of Subtypes of Gastrointestinal Vagal Afferents', *Front Physiol.* 2020 Jun 11; 11: 643.

Chapter 14: 'Naturally lean' secrets

Dunn C, Haubenreiser M, Johnson M, Nordby K, Aggarwal S, Myer S, Thomas C, 'Mindfulness approaches and weight loss, weight maintenance, and weight regain', *Curr Obes Rep.* 2018 Mar; 7 (1): 37–49.

Edmund, M, *Edison.* (New York: Random House, 2020).

Erskine, RG, 'Life Scripts: Unconscious Relational Patterns and Psychotherapeutic Involvement'. In *Life Scripts: A Transactional Analysis of Unconscious Relational Patterns* (New York: Routledge, 2018), 1–28.

Hales SD and Johnson JA, 'Dispositional optimism and luck attributions: Implications for philosophical theories of luck', *Philosophical Psychology* 2018 Jul; 31 (7): 1027–45.

Kokkinos A, le Roux CW, Alexiadou K, Tentolouris N, Vincent RP, Kyriaki D, Perrea D, Ghatei MA, Bloom SR, Katsilambros N, 'Eating slowly increases the postprandial response of the anorexigenic gut hormones, peptide YY and glucagon-like peptide-1', *J Clin Endocrinol Metab.* 2010 Jan; 95 (1): 333–7.

Lean ME and Malkova D, 'Altered gut and adipose tissue hormones in overweight and obese individuals: cause or consequence?' *Int J Obes (Lond).* 2016 Apr; 40 (4): 622–32.

Levine JA, Eberhardt NL, Jensen MD, 'Role of nonexercise activity thermogenesis in resistance to fat gain in humans', *Science* 1999 Jan 8; 283 (5399): 212–14.

Levine JA, Lanningham-Foster LM, McCrady SK, Krizan AC, Olson LR, Kane PH, Jensen MD, Clark MM, 'Interindividual variation in posture allocation: possible role in human obesity', *Science* 2005 Jan 28; 307 (5709): 584–6.

Library of Congress: *Life of Thomas Alva Edison*. Library of Congress, Washington DC. Available at: https://www.loc.gov/collections/edison-company-motion-pictures-and-sound-recordings/articles-and-essays/biography/life-of-thomas-alva-edison/

Maruyama K, Sato S, Ohira T, Maeda K, Noda H, Kubota Y, Nishimura S, Kitamura A, Kiyama M, Okada T, Imano H, Nakamura M, Ishikawa Y, Kurokawa M, Sasaki S, Iso H, 'The joint impact on being overweight of self reported behaviours of eating quickly and eating until full: cross sectional survey', *BMJ* 2008 Oct 21; 337: a2002.

Shakespeare W, *As You Like It* (London: Penguin Classics, 2015).

Thomas EL, Frost G, Taylor-Robinson SD, Bell JD, 'Excess body fat in obese and normal-weight subjects', *Nutr Res Rev.* 2012 Jun; 25 (1): 150–61.

Traeger L, 'Catastrophizing/Catastrophic Thinking'. In *Encyclopedia of Behavioral Medicine*, ed. Gellman MD, Turner JR (New York: Springer, 2013).

Wooden J, *Wooden: A Lifetime of Observations and Reflections On and Off the Court* (McGraw-Hill, 1997).

Index